MILADY STANDARD COSMETOLOGY:

Haircoloring and Chemical Texture Services

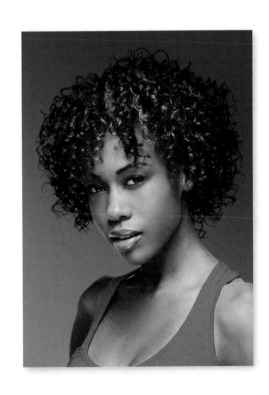

MILADY STANDARD COSMETOLOGY:

Haircoloring and Chemical Texture Services

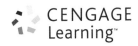

CENGAGE
Learning™

Australia • Brazil • Japan • Korea • Mexico • Singapore • Spain • United Kingdom • United States

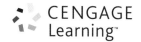
CENGAGE
Learning™

Milady Standard Cosmetology: Haircoloring and Chemical Texture Services
Colleen Hennessey, Victoria Wurdinger

President, Milady: Dawn Gerrain

Director of Content and Business Development: Sandra Bruce

Associate Acquisitions Editor: Philip Mandl

Product Manager: Maria Moffre-Barnes

Editorial Assistant: Elizabeth A. Edwards

Director of Marketing and Training: Gerard McAvey

Marketing Manager: Matthew McGuire

Senior Production Director: Wendy A. Troeger

Production Manager: Sherondra Thedford

Senior Content Project Manager: Angela Sheehan

Technology Director: Sandy Charette

Senior Art Director: Benjamin Gleeksman

Title page photo © Bruce Talbot/DK Stock/ Corbis

For product information and technology assistance, contact us at
Cengage Learning Customer & Sales Support, 1-800-354-9706

For permission to use material from this text or product,
submit all requests online at **www.cengage.com/permissions**
Further permissions questions can be emailed to
permissionrequest@cengage.com

ISBN-13: 978-1-4390-5894-7

ISBN-10: 1-4390-5894-6

Milady
Executive Woods
5 Maxwell Drive
Clifton Park, NY 12065
USA

Cengage Learning is a leading provider of customized learning solutions with office locations around the globe, including Singapore, the United Kingdom, Australia, Mexico, Brazil, and Japan. Locate your local office at **www.cengage.com/global**

Cengage Learning products are represented in Canada by Nelson Education, Ltd.

To learn more about Milady, visit **milady.cengage.com**

Purchase any of our products at your local college store or at our preferred online store **www.cengagebrain.com**

Printed in China
4 5 6 7 17 16 15 14

Table of Contents

Preface

Milady Standard Cosmetology: Haircoloring and Chemical Texture Services is a full-color, spiral-bound supplement to the leading cosmetology textbook, *Milady Standard Cosmetology*. This workbook provides you with step-by-step technical procedures for Haircoloring and Chemical Texture Services. Each technical element features two components: an overview and procedure. The overview is a short introduction providing a framework about the technique you will learn. The procedure is the step-by-step section of the technique. Each step is explained in detail and is accompanied throughout by photos. Many of the techniques will also have a variation of the technique. Each technique will include a before procedure photo and after procedure finished shot. All procedures end with photos of the same technique performed on different hair lengths, colors, and textures to help ignite your imagination. This will help you consider different possibilities for applying what you've learned in many creative ways.

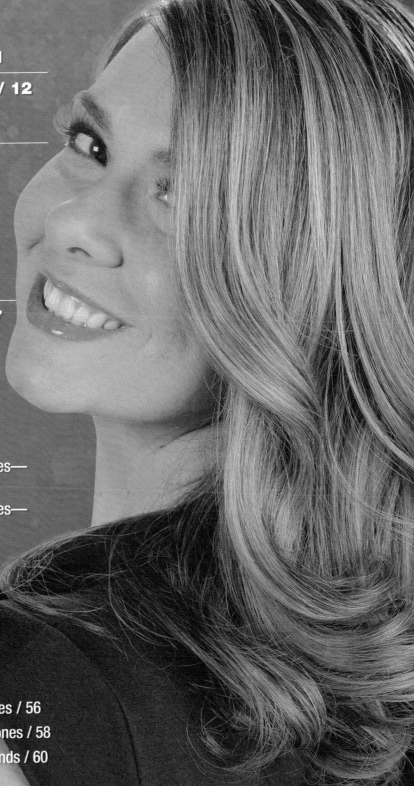

HAIRCOLORING

Introduction

Haircolor Guidelines

As we continue our study of haircolor, we must realize that it is one of the most frequently asked for services in the salon and one of the most lucrative skills a cosmetologist can master. Haircoloring provides us a unique opportunity to change how a person looks and feels about their self in a very short time. It is the ultimate cosmetic for the hair!

The basic principles of what a haircolor product does are simple:

- It provides color that lasts from shampoo to shampoo.

- It deposits color.

- It lightens and deposits new tone.

- It can remove artificial or natural pigment from the hair.

During your cosmetology career it is important to understand some key fundamental principles, which are referred to as the *Colorist Code of Conduct*, for successful haircoloring. These principles will help you master your skill level and leverage your haircolor ability. Becoming a successful colorist takes time, practice, and patience.

Before we begin any haircolor service, let's take a look at the steps involved in the *Colorist Code of Conduct*.

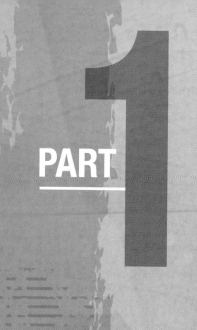

© oksana2010/www.Shutterstock.com

Colorist Code of Conduct

1. Hair Examination

2. Identifying Level

3. Identifying Tone

4. Consultation

5. Type of Haircolor Service Performed

6. Formulation/Technical Platform

7. Assessing and Applying

8. Color Removal

9. Color Results and Home-Maintenance

1 Hair Examination

- Examine the hair from the scalp area to the shaft to the ends.
- Has the hair been previously colored? If yes, prepare a plan to control what has been previously done.
- Is the hair porous?
- Remember, the more damaged and porous the hair, the darker and cooler the haircolor result can be.
- Consider the natural texture of the hair. Is it coarse, medium, or fine? Hair that is coarser may require more processing time or the use of a higher volume developer.
- What is the density of the hair on the head? (How much hair is there per square inch (2.5 square cm)?) More hair per square inch (2.5 square cm) may require for the application of more color product and smaller subsections during application.

2 Identifying Level

- Determine how light or dark the current level is in the hair by using a Level Finder swatch guide.
- Is there any gray present?
- Are the ends lighter or darker?
- What is the desired level?
- Figure out how many levels of lift are required to achieve result.
- Figure out how you will deepen the hair if darker result is desired.

3 Identifying Tone

- If decolorizing the natural color, remember that contributing pigments or undertones from the natural color will be exposed when lifting natural hair color. Balance the formula by adding warmth or coolness to the formula.
- Select warm base colors to create brighter colors, such as for red or gold tones.
- Select cooler base tones to reveal less gold or warmth in the color result.
- When gray hair is present, it is advised to add a neutral base color into the formula for balanced results.

4 Consultation

- Listen to what the client is saying.
- Read between the lines. Show photos of different colors for a visual guide.
- Ask questions.
- Suggest at least two different haircolor options with pricing.
- Don't overpromise.
- Ask what they like about their current hair color.
- Ask what they don't like about their current hair color.

5 Type of Haircolor Service Performed

- Will all-over color be applied?
- Will highlights or lowlights wrapped in foil be applied?
- Will color be applied to the regrowth only?
- Do the ends need to be refreshed?

Introduction continued

6 Formulation/Technical Platform

- Know the limits of what you can and can't do.
- Understand all the color product lines you use.
- Know the difference between haircolor lines such as depth of levels, etc.
- Compare the intensity or strength of tones.
- Know when to adjust formulas lighter and warmer for hair that is overly porous or compromised.
- Remember to take a visual picture of the starting level and the haircolor applied, so you have a mental snapshot and can train your eye to remember the haircolor that was created.
- Record all the formulas, timing, and results.

7 Assessing and Applying

- Evaluate the condition of the hair before beginning the service.
- Pay attention to the product choices to achieve results.
- Select the haircolor tools for the service.
- Beware of your application skills.
- Be neat when you are applying.
- Be sure to clean around the hairline at the end of each application.

8 Color Removal

- Rinse the color from the head by starting at the hairline and work the color through.
- Rinse until the water runs clear. Make sure you remove the color at the nape of the neck.
- When removing foils, pull one foil out at a time. Start adding some water and rinse each one. Once all the foils are removed, rinse the whole head.
- When working with color that is placed in-between foils, pull the foils out one at a time and rinse the colored sections in-between at the same time.
- Be sure to shampoo the hair so all the color is removed.
- Use a stain remover around the hairline to remove any stains.
- Use a color-preserving conditioner to add moisture to the hair and seal in the color.

9 Color Results and Home-Maintenance

- Review the color result with the client to make sure they are satisfied.
- Recommend a shampoo and conditioner to help extend the color service.
- Review and schedule a follow-up appointment.

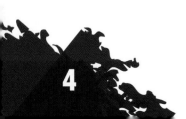

4

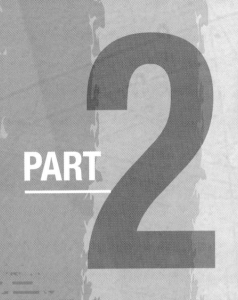

PART 2

Mixing

Learning to mix haircolor is a very important skill. There are several haircolor manufacturers that provide a wide range of products to choose from. It is important to read and review the mixing instructions for all products before you begin.

Review the *Colorist Code of Conduct* for mixing:

- Read the manufacturer's directions.

- Use clean, disinfected tools.

- Measure accurately.

- Mix until the desired consistency is reached.

- Work neatly.

Most haircolor mixtures combine a color and a developer:

- 1:1 mixing ratio refers to equal parts of color and equal parts of developer.

- 1:2 mixing ratio refers to one part color and two parts developer.

- Most high-lift blond formulas use the 1:2 ratio converted to a formula that would read: 1 ounce (30 ml) high-lift blond color to 2 ounces (60 ml) of developer.

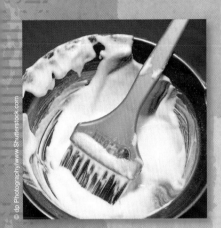

Lighteners are mixed differently than haircolor products. Some require activators mixed into the formula. These activators provide more lifting action during the color service. Other lightning products are powder for off-scalp use. These are mixed in a bowl until a creamy consistency is reached.

Applicator Bottle (1:1 Ratio)

Implements and Materials

You will need all of the following implements, materials, and supplies:

- **Towels**
- **Haircolor**
- **Hydrogen peroxide developer**
- **Applicator bottle**
- **Gloves**

Overview

In the following procedural steps you will mix combinations of different products.

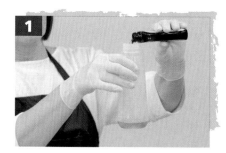

1 Pour 2 ounces (60 ml) of the color into the applicator bottle.

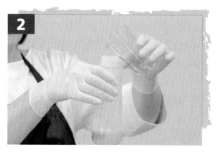

2 Add 2 ounces (60 ml) of the developer.

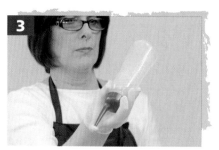

3 Put the top on the bottle and shake gently until mixed.

Applicator Bottle (1:2 Ratio)

Implements and Materials

You will need all of the following implements, materials, and supplies:

- Towels
- Haircolor
- Hydrogen peroxide developer
- Applicator bottle
- Gloves

Overview

In the following procedural steps you will mix combinations of different products.

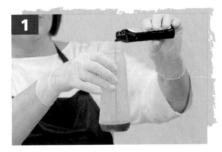

1 Here, 1:2 mixing is shown for a high-lift color formula. Pour 2 ounces (60 ml) of color into the applicator bottlc.

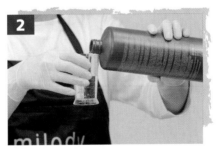

2 Add 4 ounces (120 ml) of developer into the bottle.

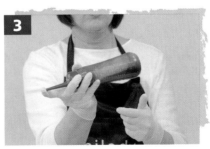

3 Put the top on the bottle and mix gently and thoroughly.

Bowl and Brush (1:1 Ratio)

Implements and Materials

You will need all of the following implements, materials, and supplies:

- **Towels**
- **Haircolor**
- **Hydrogen peroxide developer**
- **Bowl**
- **Haircolor brush**
- **Gloves**
- **Haircolor wisk**

Overview

In the following procedural steps you will mix combinations of different products.

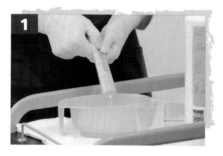

1 Pour 2 ounces (60 ml) of color into the bowl.

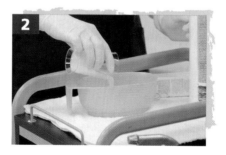

2 Measure 2 ounces (60 ml) of developer into an applicator bottle. Pour into the bowl with the color.

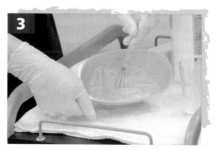

3 Mix to a creamy consistency.

On-the-Scalp Lighteners in Applicator Bottle or Bowl (2:1 Ratio)

Implements and Materials

You will need all of the following implements, materials, and supplies:

- Towels
- On-the-scalp lightener
- Hydrogen peroxide developer
- Applicator bottle
- Bowl
- Haircolor brush
- Gloves
- Haircolor wisk

Overview

In the following procedural steps you will mix combinations of different products. Pictured below is the On-the-Scalp Lightener being mixed in a bow.

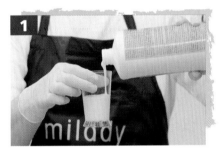

1 Pour 4 ounces (120 ml) of 20-volume developer into the applicator bottle or bowl.

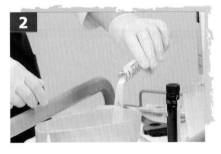

2 Add one to three lightening activators according to the amount of lightening desired. Follow the manufacturer directions.

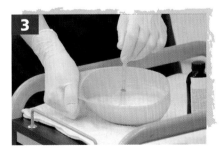

3 Put top on the bottle and shake gently or wisk lightener to desired consistency.

On-the-Scalp Lighteners in Applicator Bottle or Bowl (2:1 Ratio) continued

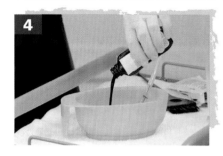

4 Add 2 ounces (60 ml) of lightener to the bottle or bowl.

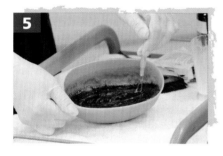

5 Put the top on the bottle and shake gently or wisk lightener to desired consistency.

Off-the-Scalp Powder Lighteners in Bowl

Implements and Materials

You will need all of the following implements, materials, and supplies:

- **Towels**
- **Off-the-scalp lightener.**
- **Hydrogen peroxide developer**
- **Bowl**
- **Haircolor brush**
- **Gloves**

Overview

In the following procedural steps you will mix combinations of different products.

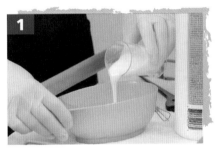

1 Pour 2 ounces (60 ml) of developer into a nonmetallic bowl.

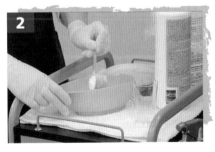

2 Add 3 to 4 scoops of powder lightener to the bowl.

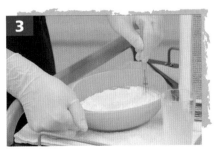

3 Mix to creamy consistency.

PART 3

Demipermanent Haircolor

Demipermanent haircolor may be the perfect solution for the client who wants to enhance their natural color without long-term commitment. You can also use demipermanent haircolor to blend gray hair, or as a color enhancement for hair that has been chemically relaxed, permed, or keratin smoothed.

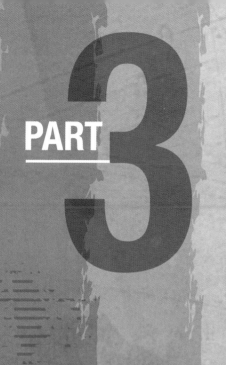

© iStockphoto/emreogan

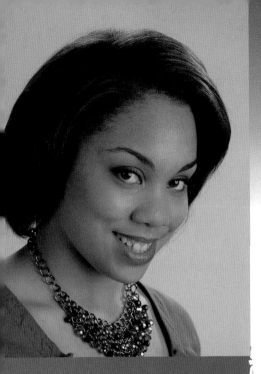

Color Enhancement for Relaxed, Permed, or Keratin Smoothed Hair

Implements and Materials

You will need all of the following implements, materials, and supplies:

- **Towels**
- **Haircolor**
- **Developer, if required**
- **Chemical cape**
- **Gloves**
- **Clips**
- **Comb**
- **Protective cream**
- **Applicator bottle**
- **Bowl and brush**
- **Timer**
- **Client service record card**
- **Color chart**

Overview

Color enhancements add tone and shine in one easy step to any hair color—without lightening the hair. A color enhancement may complement a wide variety of hair colors, whether blond, red, brunette, or black. The total color service takes about 30 minutes. Color-enhancement services and relaxers can be done successfully on the same day with nonammonia coloring products.

Mastering color enhancements will build a strong foundation for other haircolor situations you will encounter. Refer to the *Colorist Code of Conduct* before you begin the color-enhancement service. Learning proper formulation and application skills is very important.

Procedure

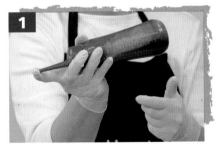

1 Mix the formula. Wear gloves when you mix and apply color.

Formula for model shown: equal parts 3RR demipermanent cream color + manufacture dedicated demipermanent color developer.

Color Enhancement for Relaxed, Permed, or Keratin Smoothed Hair continued

2 Part the hair into four sections with the tip of the applicator bottle. Apply protective cream to the hairline and ears.

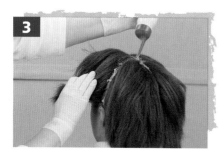

3 Outline each section of hair—from ear to ear and from front forehead to center nape—with haircolor.

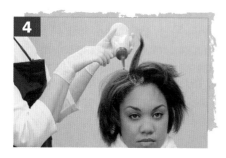

4 Begin applying where the hair is the most resistant. Here, you will start in the front right section. Take ½-inch (1.25 cm) partings and apply the color at the scalp area working neatly, precisely, and efficiently. Bring all sections out away from the head to allow air to circulate. Move to the front left section and apply color to the scalp area, again taking ½-inch (2.5 cm) partings. Continue until the section is complete.

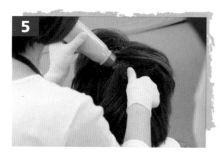

5 Move to the back sections of the head, following the same method. Work neatly until each section is completed.

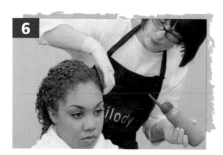

6 After color has been applied to all four sections, begin to work the color down the hair shaft to the ends, making sure the hair is saturated with color. Gently massage the color through all of the hair. Do not rub or work aggressively. Set the timer for up to 20 minutes to process the color. *

* Depending on manufacturers recommendations, rinse or shampoo color product from the hair. Condition and finish as desired.

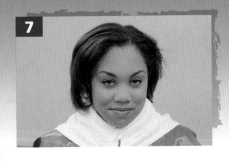

7 Before Color Enhancement for Relaxed, Permed, or Keratin Smoothed Hair Procedure.

Service Tip

Be sure to review the *Colorist Code of Conduct* for color removal to follow the proper steps. This new color accents the relaxed hair. Coloring and relaxing services can be done successfully on the same day.

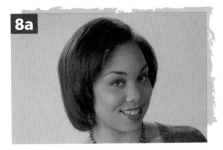

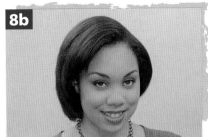

8 After Color Enhancement for Relaxed, Permed, or Keratin Smoothed Hair Procedure.

Create

Apply this technique to different hair lengths, colors, and textures for almost endless possibilities.

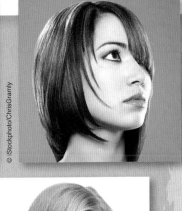
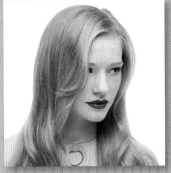
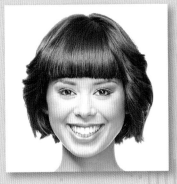
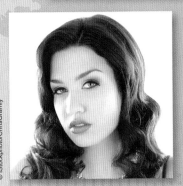

4

Permanent Haircolor

Now that you have worked with nonammonia color-enhancing products, it is time to graduate to the next phase of haircoloring: permanent haircolor. Permanent haircolor can lighten or deepen natural color, change tone, and cover gray hair—the possibilities are endless.

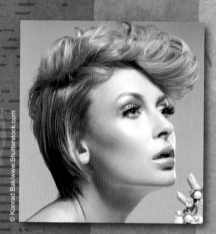

© Konrad Bak/www.Shutterstock.com

16

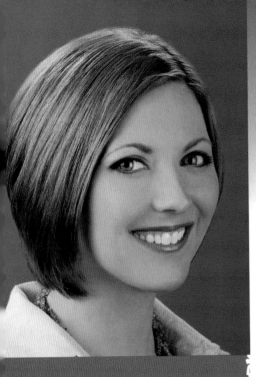

Virgin Application— Bowl and Brush

Implements and Materials

You will need all of the following implements, materials, and supplies:

- **Towels**
- **Haircolor**
- **Developer**
- **Chemical cape**
- **Gloves**
- **Clips**
- **Comb**
- **Bowl and brush**
- **Timer**
- **Client service record card**
- **Color chart**

Overview

You will begin permanent haircoloring by lightening natural pigment. This is referred to as a *virgin application going lighter*. It is a popular service with clients who want to lighten and change the tone of their existing color. Before you begin this service, you must review the Colorist Code of Conduct.

Next, examine the hair to determine its condition and answer these three important questions before beginning the haircolor service:

1. What is the level of the natural hair? (Remember to assess the scalp area, shaft, and ends.)

2. What is the desired end level and tone that the client wishes?

3. What formulation will achieve the desired results?

Once these questions are answered, you can mix the formula and determine which application method you will be using to apply the color. In the following examples of permanent color, you will see demonstrated the use of an applicator bottle and a bowl and brush.

Procedure

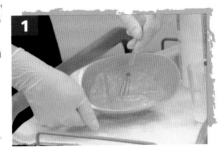

1 Put on gloves and mix the color formula.

Formula: The formula used on our model—1½ parts 8GN + ½ part 8A permanent cream color + 2 parts 20-volume manufacture dedicated developer.

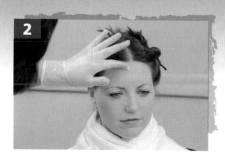

2 Part the hair into four sections—from ear to ear and straight down the back of the head. Apply protective cream to the hairline and ears.

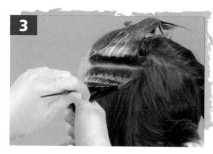

3 Begin the section where the color change will be greatest or where the hair is most resistant, usually the hairline and temple areas. Part off a ¼-inch (.6 cm) subsection with the tail of the applicator brush. Lift the subsection and apply color to the mid-strand area. Stay at least ½ inch (1.25 cm) from the scalp and do not apply to the porous ends.

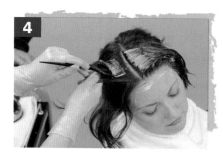

4 Continue around the head with the same application technique using the bowl and brush.

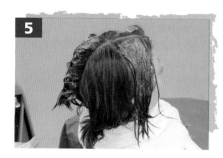

5 Apply the color to the back of the head taking ¼-inch (.6 cm) subsections and applying ½ inch (1.25 cm) away from the scalp.

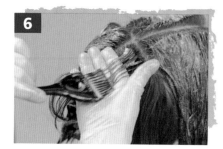

6 Work precisely and quickly through each section. Use the brush and the fingers to work the color formula into the hair.

Part 1: Haircoloring

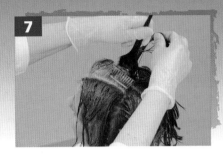

7 Next, complete the fourth quadrant. Separate the hair to aerate, allowing for oxidation.

8 Continue the application process down to the nape hairline area. Where lengths are extremely short in this area, work color throughout.

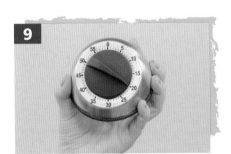

9 Process according to the strand test results (for half of the total processing time). Check for color development by removing color as described in the strand test procedure.

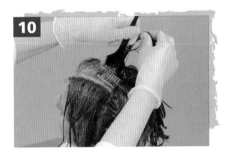

10 Now apply the color to the scalp area in all four sections. Outline the quadrants first.

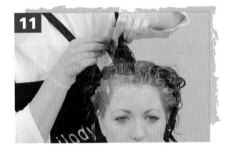

11 Take ¼-inch (.6 cm) subsections, applying color to the ½-inch (1.25 cm) area at the scalp and working color through each subsection until the head is completed. Work the color through the ends of the hair. Work neatly and efficiently, making sure to apply enough color to thoroughly saturate the hair, including around the front hairline.

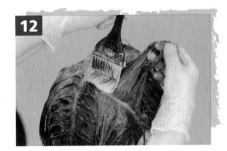

12 Work through the interior of the back quadrants using the brush method.

Virgin Application—Bowl and Brush continued

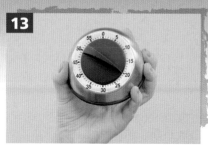

13 Set the timer for the additional time needed. Most processing time is 45 minutes.*

* Depending on manufacturers recommendations, rinse or shampoo color product from the hair. Condition and finish as desired.

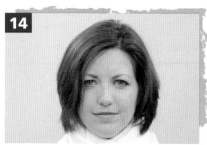

14 Before Permanent Haircolor: Virgin Application—Bowl and Brush Procedure.

Service Tip

Follow the *Colorist Code of Conduct* for color removal

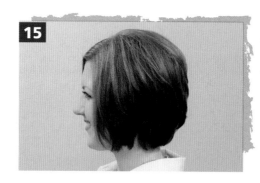

15 After Permanent Haircolor: Virgin Application—Bowl and Brush Procedure.

Create

Apply this technique to different hair lengths, colors, and textures for almost endless possibilities.

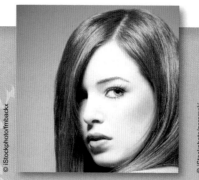

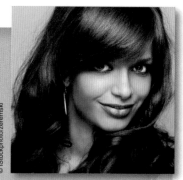

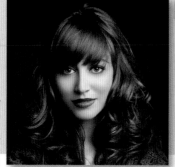

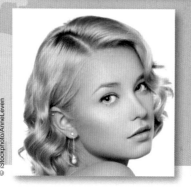

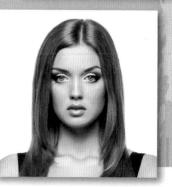

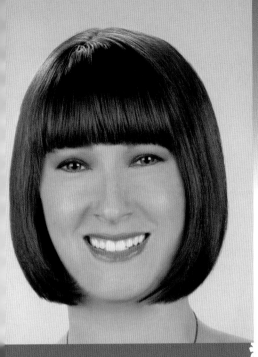

Covering Gray— Applicator Bottle

Implements and Materials

You will need all of the following implements, materials, and supplies:

- **Towels**
- **Haircolor**
- **Developer**
- **Chemical cape**
- **Gloves**
- **Clips**
- **Comb**
- **Applicator Bottle**
- **Timer**
- **Client service record card**
- **Color chart**

Overview

Gray hair is still the number one reason why people color their hair. To cover gray completely, your best choice is a permanent haircolor—but there are different ways to change gray hair to suit the client.

Understanding the difference between *blending* and *covering* gray hair is the key to a successful consultation. When a client sees that they are faced with a few gray hairs, they usually want to get rid of them. They will say things like, "Can I try a color?" or, "Can I make the gray hair look highlighted?" This is when you should reach for a nonammonia color to blend the gray. This type of color service has more sheer results, and it will also wash out faster, meaning it is less permanent. Keep in mind, when using a nonammonia color, that it will not lighten the natural color and will focus more on blending the gray.

Once the client starts seeing more than just a few gray hairs, however, he or she is usually looking to get rid of them completely. Now you should reach for a permanent color to cover the gray. Remember that since permanent color can lighten, you will be able to create a softer gray coverage look by slightly lightening the pigmented hair and adding color to the gray.

Here are some gray coverage tips to remember before you formulate and start your color service:

- Formulate a gray coverage formula by staying two levels lighter than the pigmented hair. For example, if the client was a Level 3 medium-brown, formulate no lighter than a Level 5 lightest-brown for a natural result.

- Use a neutral tone alone or mix it with an ash, red, or gold base with 20-volume developer.

Covering Gray—Applicator Bottle continued

- Formulate at a Level 8 light-blond and deeper for your best coverage result.

- Process the color for a full 45 minutes.

- If you are working with resistant gray hair add ½ ounce (15 ml) of a deeper color to the formula.

- Take fine, even sections and saturate the hair completely.

Remember to review the *Colorist Code of Conduct* for Haircolor before you begin any color service.

Procedure

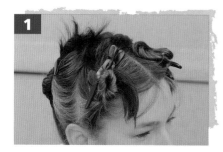

1 Part the hair into four sections—from ear to ear and straight down the back of the head. Put on gloves and mix the color formula. Apply protective cream to the hairline and ears.

> **Formula:** The formula used on our model—1 part 3G + 1 part 4G + ½ part 4RO + ½ part 3RV + permanent color + 3 parts 30-volume manufacture dedicated developer.

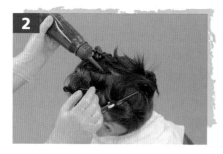

2 Outline all four sections with color beginning with the center front section then move to the sides.

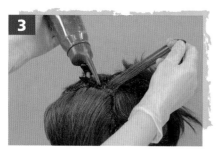

3 Next using ¼-inch (.6 cm) diagonal subsections, apply the color to the scalp area.

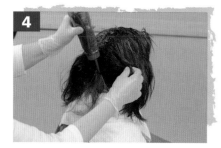

4 Continue around the head using ¼-inch (.6 cm) diagonal subsections.

5 Once all four sections are complete, work the rest of the color through to the ends. Process the color for 45 minutes, or according to the manufacturer's directions.*

* Depending on manufacturers recommendations, rinse or shampoo color product from the hair. Condition and finish as desired.

6 Record all formulas and recommended specific shampoos and conditioners for color-treated hair. Notice how one simple formula can make a client look more youthful.

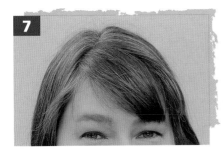

7 Before Permanent Haircolor: Covering Gray—Applicator Bottle Procedure.

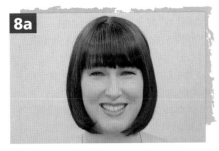

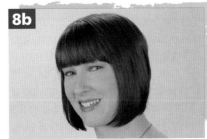

8 After Permanent Haircolor: Covering Gray—Applicator Bottle Procedure.

Create

Apply this technique to different hair lengths, colors, and textures for almost endless possibilities.

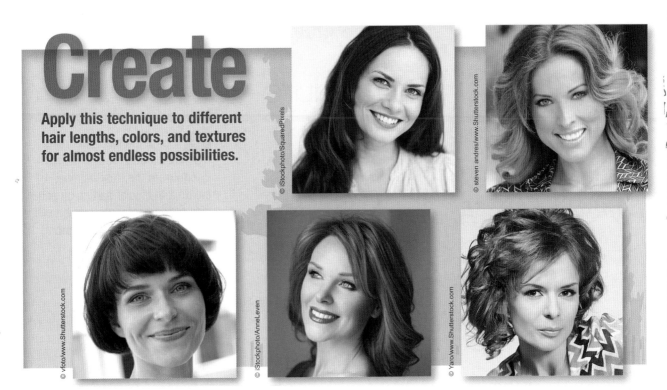

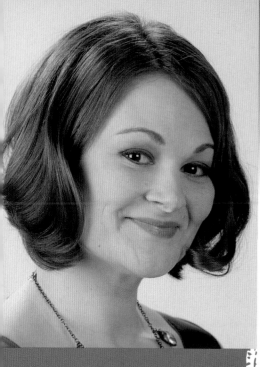

Block Color—Bowl and Brush

Implements and Materials

You will need all of the following implements, materials, and supplies:

- **Towels**
- **Haircolor**
- **Developer**
- **Chemical cape**
- **Gloves**
- **Clips**
- **Comb**
- **Bowl and brush**
- **Timer**
- **Client service record card**
- **Color chart**

Overview

By now you understand that when permanent color is used, you can make many changes with haircolor. The *Block Color Technique* is a simple technique using two different formulas placed on the head to create subtle or dramatic changes, depending on the color formulas you choose. This technique is done by making a diamond-shape parting on the top of the head and a zigzag parting from the occipital bone across from ear to ear. One color formulation is placed in these two blocked-off sections, while a second formula is applied to the rest of the hair. The creative results are endless with this technique.

Refer to the *Colorist Code of Conduct* for Haircolor before you begin.

Procedure

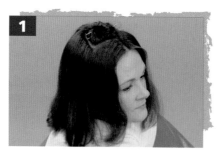

1 Comb the hair and create a center parting. Now, 2 inches (5 cm) from the front hairline, create a triangular parting on either side of the center part, which will create a diamond-shape parting across the top of the head.

2 Once you've completed the shape, clip the hair up and out of the way.

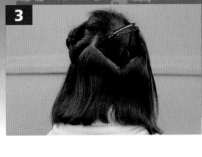

3 Go to the back of the head from ear to ear and make a zigzag parting across the back of the head slightly above the occipital bone.

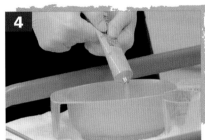

4 Select the two formulas. For example, if you select two red colors, one can be light and very bright and the other can be deeper to create a vivid contrast.

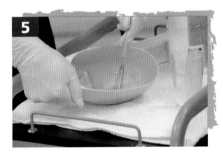

5 Put on gloves and mix the two formulas in separate bowls. Apply protective cream to the hairline and ears.

The formula used on our model:

- Diamond and the nape: 2 parts 3RR permanent cream color + 2 parts 20-volume manufacture dedicated developer.
- Remainder of Head: 2 parts 6RO permanent cream color + 2 parts 20-volume manufacture dedicated developer.

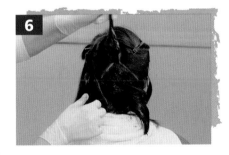

6 Begin by outlining the zigzag area with Formula 1, then apply Formula 1 to the outlined area below the occipital bone throughout the nape. Move to the left side and apply Formula 1 to the diamond-shaped section by first outlining it with color, and then by taking fine sections and applying the formula from the roots to the ends. When the section is completed, clip it up.

7 Repeat on the right side. Once the diamond section has color applied, clip out of the way.

Block Color—Bowl and Brush continued

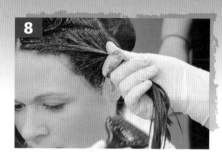

8 Take Formula 2 and apply it from scalp area to ends of the uncolored areas remaining around the head.

9 Process the color for 30 minutes.

10 Rinse the color with warm water. Take down the two blocks and rinse first. Then add the rest of the hair. Shampoo and condition hair.

11 Style and review the color results.

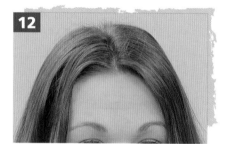

12 Before Permanent Haircolor: Block Color—Bowl and Brush Procedure.

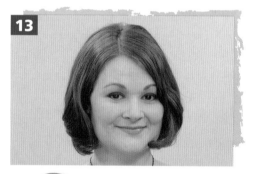

13 After Permanent Haircolor: Block Color—Bowl and Brush Procedure.

Create

Apply this technique to different hair lengths, colors, and textures for almost endless possibilities.

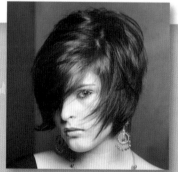
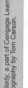
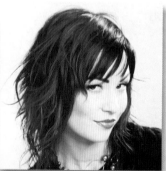
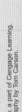
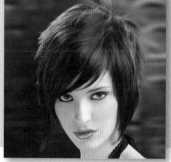
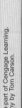
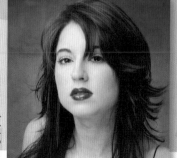
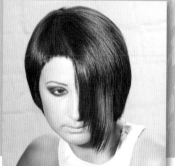

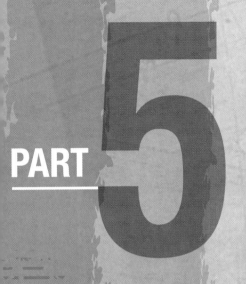

PART 5

Dimensional Haircolor Services

Dimensional haircolor services—better known as *highlighting*—is one of the fastest-growing haircolor markets. This is where your creativity can be endless.

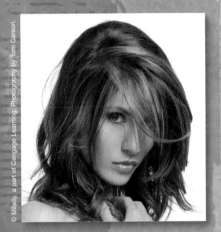

Foiling is the professional choice for highlighting the hair. It provides tremendous control in the application and creates precision results. Here you will learn some of the most popular techniques used in the salon today. We will focus on some different foil-wrapping methods: face-frame highlight with a single-process color application between the foils; partial highlight; a retouch highlight; and how to place some interesting accent pieces.

You will also learn the difference between slicing and weaving, and see how each affects the result.

Review the *Colorist Code of Conduct* before you begin the haircolor service.

© Milady, a part of Cengage Learning. Photography by Tom Carson.

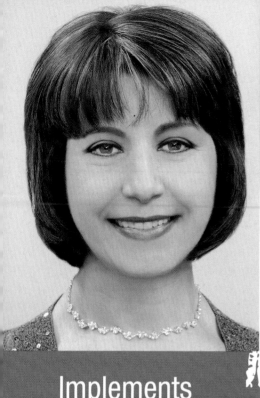

Face-Frame with Single-Process Color

Implements and Materials

You will need all of the following implements, materials, and supplies:

- Towels
- Haircolor
- Lightener
- Developer
- Chemical cape
- Gloves
- Foils
- Clips
- Comb
- Applicator bottle
- Bowl and brush
- Foil tip comb
- Timer
- Client service record card
- Color chart

Overview

In this service you will simultaneously perform a face-framing highlight and single-process color.

Procedure

Formula: Lightener—an off-the-scalp lightener with a neutral color base was used to lighten the hair. This product was mixed to the desired consistency with the manufacture dedicated 20-volume developer.

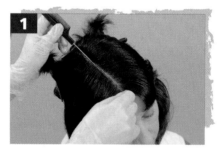

1 Begin by putting on gloves, mixing the two color formulas and, using a tail or foil tip comb, part the hair into four sections.

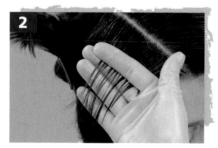

2 Beginning at the right of the part, part out a slice of hair with the tail or foil tip comb.

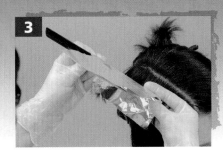

3 While holding the slice of hair, pick up a piece of foil. Fold the foil over the comb.

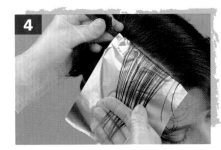

4 Lay the hair on top of the foil, getting as close to the scalp as possible.

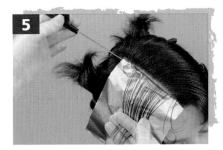

5 Next, slide the comb out from underneath the foil and hold the hair taut to the foil.

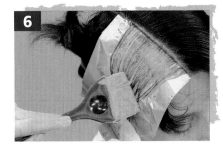

6 Next, brush on the highlighting color product starting at the top of the foil and working the product down the strand.

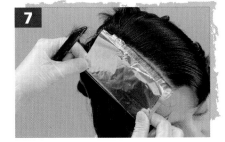

7 Fold the foil in half to meet the piece at the top.

Face-Frame with Single-Process Color

continued

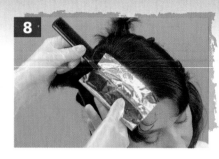

8 With the metal end of your comb, crease the center of the foil.

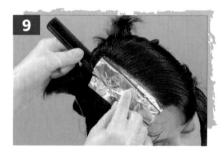

9 Fold the foil again and slide the metal end of your comb out.

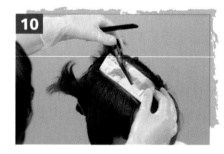

10 Clip the foil up and out of the way.

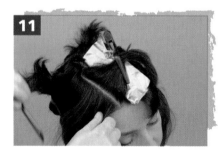

11 Part out ½-inch (1.25 cm) subsection of hair in-between each foiled slice.

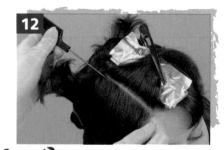

12 Clip each foil section up and out of the way.

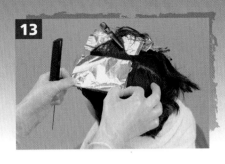

13 Continue working down the side in the same way. The foils on the side will go to the temple area. Once the section is complete, move to the opposite side of the part and complete that section. Start this section by parting out a ½-inch (1.25 cm) subsection; this section will not be in a foil. Then continue the foiling process using ⅛-inch (.3 cm) slices and ½-inch (1.25 cm) subsections in-between the slices.

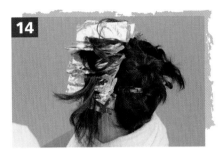

14 Here, all the foils are in.

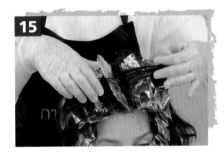

15 Once the foils are securely placed, you are ready to color the hair in-between the foils.

Formula: The formula used on our model—1 part 4RN + 1 part 6G permanent cream color + 2 parts 20-volume manufacture dedicated developer.

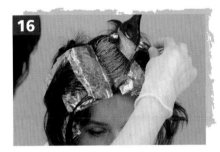

16 Start in the center of the head. Apply the second color formula to the hair that is in-between each of the foils. Apply the color at the scalp area and work it down the length of the strand until it is completely saturated.

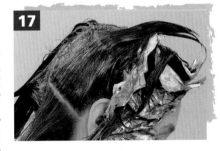

17 Continue to work in-between each foil and apply the color until the whole head is completed.

a. After the color application in the front is complete, fold the foils out of the face and apply color to the front hairline.

b. Move to the left back section, outline the section with color, then take ½-inch (1.25 cm) subsections and apply color from the scalp area to ends through the entire section. Complete the right side in the same manner. Set a timer to process.

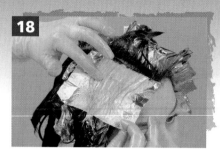

18 Open a foil to see if the color has reached the desired lightness. When complete, remove and rinse the foils one at a time, rinse hair thoroughly, then shampoo and condition. Apply a glaze if desired.

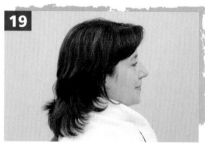

19 Before Dimensional Haircolor Services: Face-Frame with Single-Process Color Procedure.

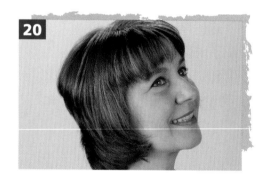

20 After Dimensional Haircolor Services: Face-Frame with Single-Process Color Procedure. Notice how this service adds a subtle amount of dimension that frames the face and intensifies the richness of the entire color.

Create

Apply this technique to different hair lengths, colors, and textures for almost endless possibilities.

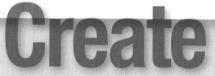
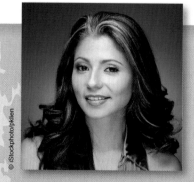
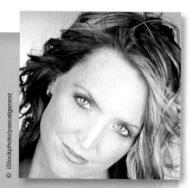
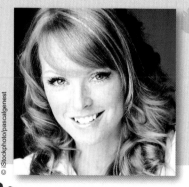
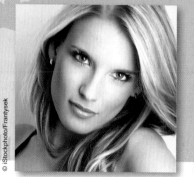
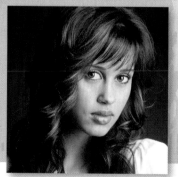

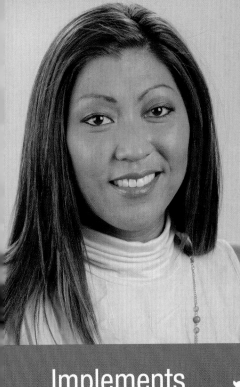

Partial Highlight

Implements and Materials

You will need all of the following implements, materials, and supplies:

- **Towels**
- **Haircolor**
- **Lightener**
- **Developer**
- **Chemical cape**
- **Gloves**
- **Foils**
- **Clips**
- **Comb**
- **Applicator bottle**
- **Bowl and brush**
- **Foil tip comb**
- **Timer**
- **Client service record card**
- **Color chart**

© Milady, a part of Cengage Learning. Photography by Gary David Gold.

Overview

In this service, you will highlight the top and sides of the head.

Procedure

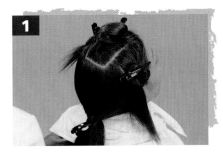

1 Begin by parting off a rectangular section on the top of the head, from middle of the eyebrow to middle of the eyebrow, and from top to side on both sides. Clip the entire back section down, out of the way.

Formula: Lightener—an off-the-scalp lightener with a neutral color base was used to lighten the hair. This product was mixed to the desired consistency with the manufacture dedicated 20-volume developer.

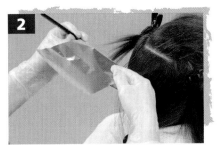

2 Take a fine ⅛-inch (.3 cm) slice starting at the crown of the head. While holding the slice of hair, pick up a piece of foil. Fold the end of the comb under the foil and place it at the scalp.

Partial Highlight continued

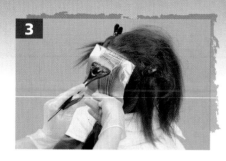

3 Brush on lightener, starting ½ inch (1.25 cm) away from the top of the foil, working the product up to the top of the foil, then down the entire strand. Double-fold the foil.

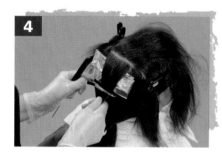

4 Release the next ½-inch (1.25 cm) section and clip out of the way. Continue working toward the front of the head.

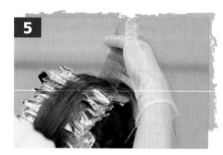

5 To create a less precise, more random look toward the front, take the metal end of your comb and weave it back and forth through the strand.

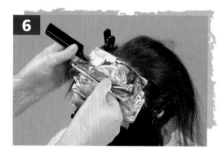

6 Slide your comb from underneath the foil. Notice the hair in the foil.

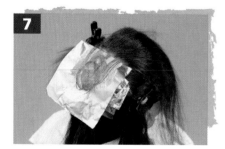

7 Apply the lightener to the hair.

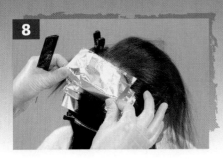

8 Bend the foil once over the hair, and then fold the foil again. Fold the foil and clip it out of the way.

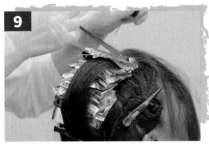

9 Part out an approximately ½-inch (1.25 cm) section to leave unfoiled, then part out a ⅛-inch (.3 cm) section for the next foil.

a. When you are 2 inches (5 cm) from the front hairline, place two ⅛-inch (.3 cm) sliced foils back-to-back to add a bolder panel of color.

b. Complete the front section by alternating ⅛-inch (.3 cm) slices in foil with ½-inch (1.25 cm) sections left out of foil up to the front hairline.

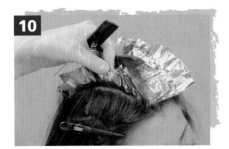

10 The top of the head is complete. It is now time to do the sides.

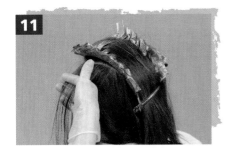

11 Take a fine ⅛-inch (.3 cm) slice at the top section of the left side.

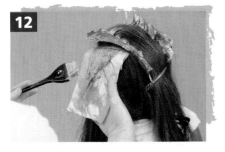

12 After placing the foil, apply the lightener, working down the entire strand.

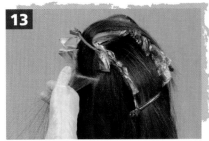

13 Clip the foil up and out of the way. Clip a section out of the way between each foil.

Part 1: Haircoloring

35

Partial Highlight continued

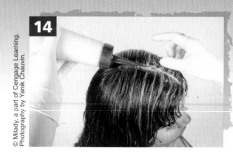

14 Complete both sides.

15 When lightener is finished processing, remove foils, rinse, and shampoo. Apply glaze if desired.

Formula: Glaze—The formula used on our model:
1 part 8N + 1 Part 7G demipermanent haircolor + 2 parts manufacture dedicated demipermanent haircolor developer.

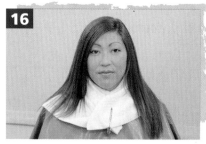

16 Before Dimensional Haircolor Services: Partial Highlight Procedure.

17 After Dimensional Haircolor Services: Partial Highlight Procedure.

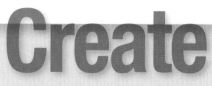

Create

Apply this technique to different hair lengths, colors, and textures for almost endless possibilities.

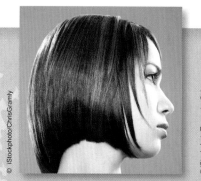

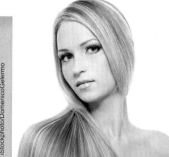

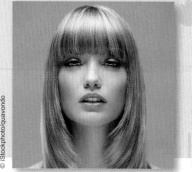

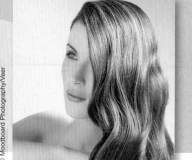

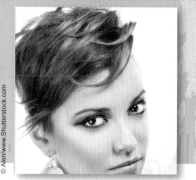

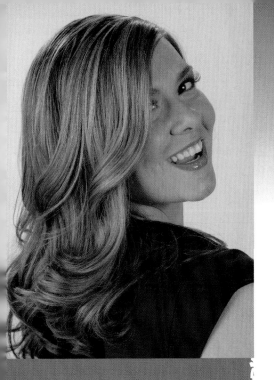

Retouch Highlight

Implements and Materials

You will need all of the following implements, materials, and supplies:

- **Towels**
- **Haircolor**
- **Lightener**
- **Developer**
- **Chemical cape**
- **Gloves**
- **Foils**
- **Clips**
- **Comb**
- **Applicator bottle**
- **Bowl and brush**
- **Foil tip comb**
- **Timer**
- **Client service record card**
- **Color chart**

Overview

A retouch highlight is a way to add highlights for a client who has already received highlights in the past. It is a way to separate previously highlighted hair so that the lightener isn't pulled through to the ends every time, resulting in overly blond hair.

Procedure

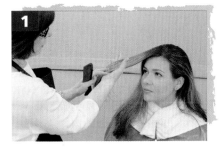

1 Consult with your client regarding her hair color wishes. Put on gloves and mix lightener. Section and clip the hair on the top of the head, out of the way.

Formula: Lightener—an off-the-scalp lightener with a neutral color base was used to lighten the hair. This product was mixed to the desired consistency with the manufacture dedicated 20-volume developer.

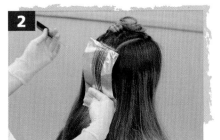

2 Now, take a slice of hair at the lower crown area of the head. Place foil under the slice.

Retouch Highlight continued

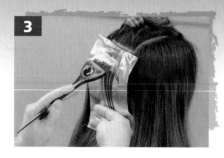

3 Holding the hair taut, brush lightener onto the new growth of the hair and place the rest of the hair out of the foil.

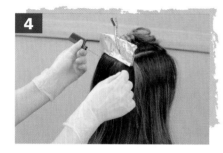

4 Double fold the foil and clip up and out of the way.

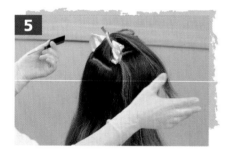

5 Take a ¾-inch (3.75 cm) subsection in-between the foils.

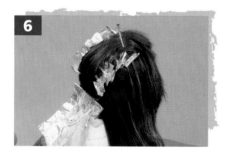

6 Continue working down the back center of the head until the section is complete. Note the contrast in size between the foiled and unfoiled sections. If hair is dark on the entire strand, apply lightener throughout.

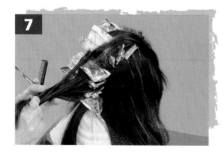

7 Once the section is complete, release the clipped-up foil and bend the ends up and out of the way on both sides of the foiled sections.

Part 1: Haircoloring

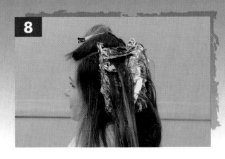

8 Working around the head, into the left side area, divide the panel into two smaller sections.

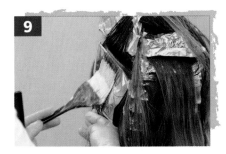

9 Work down the side panels by taking fine slices of hair and placing them into foil. Continue this process through both side panels, clipping the foils up and out of the way.

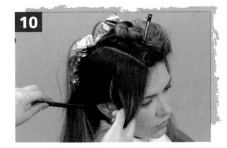

10 Move to the right side of the head and complete in the same manner.

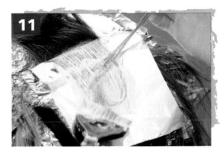

11 Now it is time to do the last section—the top of the head. Take a fine slice of hair off the top of a larger section and place it on the foil.

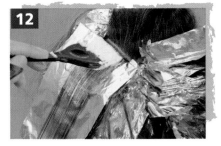

12 Apply the product to the new growth of the hair and place the rest of the hair outside of the foil.

Part 1: Haircoloring

Retouch Highlight continued

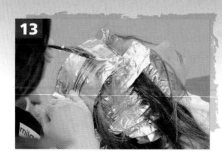

13 Part out a larger section, and then take a fine slice from the top of this section.

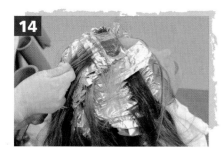

14 Continue to the front until the last foil is place. Place under a heated dryer until processes is complete, if needed.

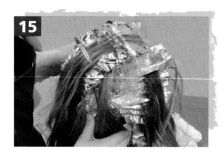

15 In this top view, you can see where the foils were placed. They were processed to a pale yellow. Note the alternation of light and dark. Once processing is completed, remove the foils, rinse, shampoo, and towel-dry.

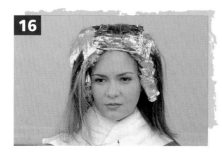

16 Apply haircolor glaze over the highlights. This will add tone and shine to the natural color and tone the highlights.

> **Formula—Glaze:** The formula used on our model: 1 part 8N + 1 part 8G demipermanent haircolor + 2 parts manufacture dedicated demipermanent haircolor developer.

17 Apply glaze all over the head in a scalp-to-ends fashion.

18 Work the color into the hair to make sure it is completely saturated. Process for 10 minutes. Rinse.*

* Depending on manufacturers recommendations, rinse or shampoo color product from the hair. Condition and finish as desired.

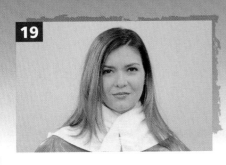

19 Before Dimensional Haircolor Services: Retouch Highlight Procedure.

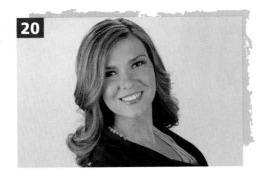

20 After Dimensional Haircolor Services: Retouch Highlight Procedure. The finished look shows beautiful golden-amber highlights all over the head. Discuss home-maintenance with the client.

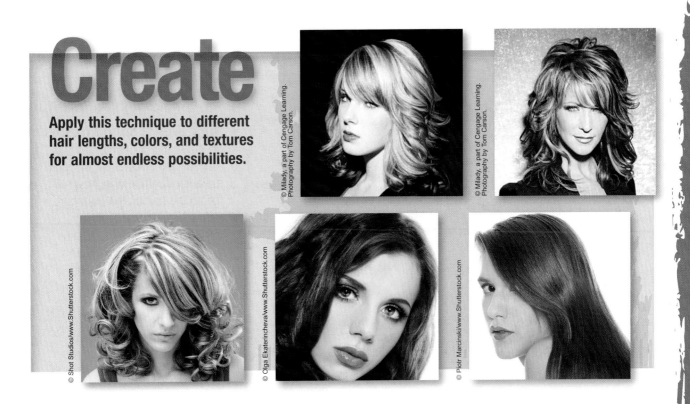

Create

Apply this technique to different hair lengths, colors, and textures for almost endless possibilities.

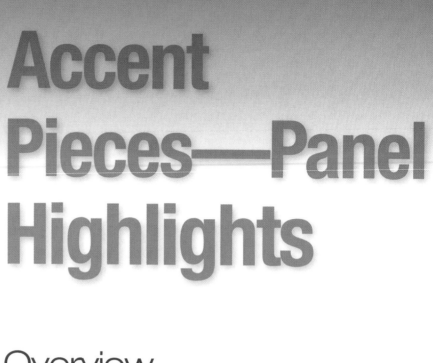

Accent Pieces—Panel Highlights

© Milady, a part of Cengage Learning. Photography by Gary David Gold.

Implements and Materials

You will need all of the following implements, materials, and supplies:

- Towels
- Haircolor
- Lightener
- Developer
- Chemical cape
- Gloves
- Foils
- Clips
- Comb
- Applicator bottle
- Bowl and brush
- Foil tip comb
- Timer
- Client service record card
- Color chart

Overview

In this service, you will create a dramatic highlight effect throughout the top portion of the head featuring wider bands of highlights.

Procedure

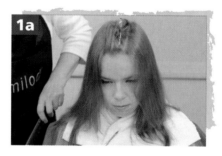

1a Begin by taking a parting from the top of the ear to top of the ear and pin the hair in, back up and out of the way. Now comb the hair on the front part of the head forward and part a 1-inch (2.5 cm) wide section down the center of the head and pin it out of the way. Put on gloves. Mix lightener.

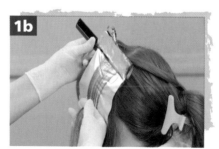

1b Starting on the left side at the crown area, take a fine diagonal slice and put it into a foil.

Formula: Lightener—an off-the-scalp lightener was used to lighten the hair. This product was mixed to the desired consistency with the manufacture dedicated 20-volume developer.

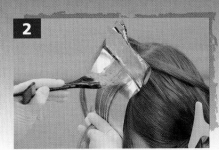

2 Apply the product to the strand and fold the foil.

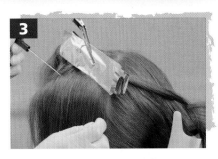

3 Without taking a subsection of hair to remain unlightened as in previous procedures, take another slice and place it right behind the first one. This will make for thick highlights that process effectively. Here you can see two foils back-to-back. Part out a 1-inch (2.5 cm) subsection to be left unlightened between the foils and work neatly and efficiently. Clip the hair not being worked on out of the way.

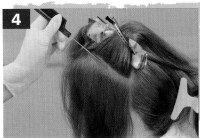

4 Part off a fine slice from the top of the section released.

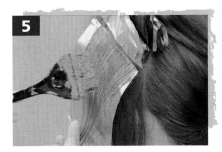

5 Place it into the foil and apply the product.

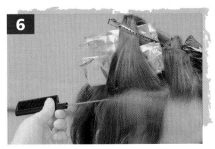

6 Continue working to the front of the head using the procedure as outlined—two fine slices foiled right next to each other with a 1-inch (2.5 cm) subsection unlightened in-between the foils.

7 Take a 1-inch (2.5 cm) subsection in-between the foils.

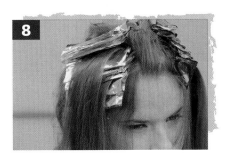

8 You can see the two foil sections back-to-back, with a 1-inch (2.5 cm) subsection in-between. Now, continue with the same procedure until you have foiled as much of the side as you desire. Move to the right side and foil the hair in the same manner.

9 Depending on manufacturers recommendations, rinse or shampoo color product from the hair. Condition and finish as desired.

Part 1: Haircoloring

Accent Pieces—Panel Highlights continued

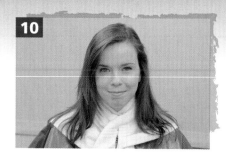

10 Before Dimensional Haircolor Services: Accent Pieces—Panel Highlights Procedure.

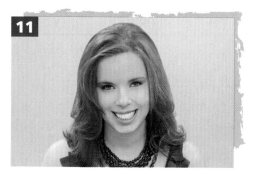

11 After Dimensional Haircolor Services: Accent Pieces—Panel Highlights Procedure. This look creates dramatic highlighted pieces of hair on the top surface of the head.

Create

Apply this technique to different hair lengths, colors, and textures for almost endless possibilities.

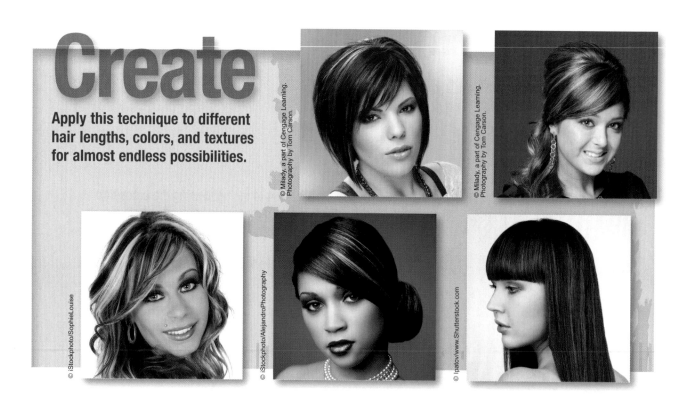

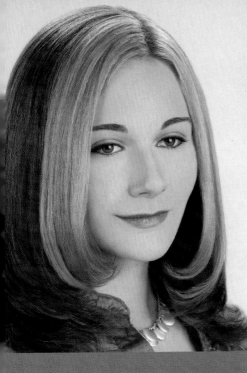

Accent Pieces—Bold Front Pieces

Implements and Materials

You will need all of the following implements, materials, and supplies:

- **Towels**
- **Haircolor**
- **Lightener**
- **Developer**
- **Chemical cape**
- **Gloves**
- **Foils**
- **Clips**
- **Comb**
- **Applicator bottle**
- **Bowl and brush**
- **Foil tip comb**
- **Timer**
- **Client service record card**
- **Color chart**

Overview

This is an easy way to add dramatic light pieces to the fringe area.

Procedure

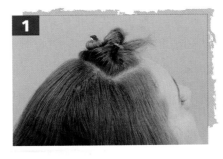

1 Part off a rectangular section from the middle of the eyebrow to the middle of the eyebrow, 1½-inches (3.75 cm) deep. Put on your gloves and mix the lightener. Take a fine slice from the back of this section and place it into the foil and apply product.

Formula: Lightener—an off-the-scalp lightener was used to lighten the hair. This product was mixed to the desired consistency with the manufacture dedicated 20-volume developer.

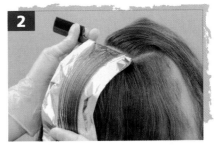

2 Double-fold the foil.

© Milady, a part of Cengage Learning. Photography by Gary David Gold.

Part 1: Haircoloring

Accent Pieces—Bold Front Pieces continued

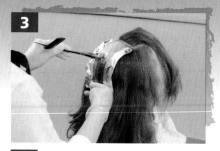

3 Take the next slice of hair back-to-back with the first one and place it onto the foil.

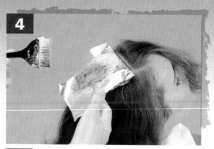

4 Continue placing foils to the front hairline. Fold the edges of the foil back to secure.

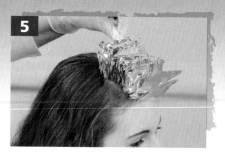

5 Here is the finished view of foils.

6 You can also tone the hair if desired.*

Formula: Glaze—1 part 6N demipermanent haircolor + 1 part manufacturer dedicated demipermanent haircolor developer.

* Depending on manufacturers recommendations, rinse or shampoo color product from the hair. Condition and finish as desired.

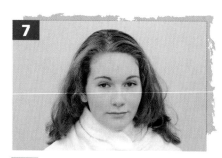

7 Before Dimensional Haircolor Services: Accent Pieces—Bold Front Pieces Procedure.

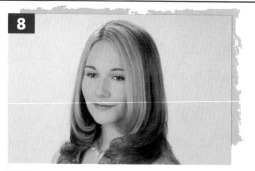

8 After Dimensional Haircolor Services: Accent Pieces—Bold Front Pieces Procedure.

Create

Apply this technique to different hair lengths, colors, and textures for almost endless possibilities.

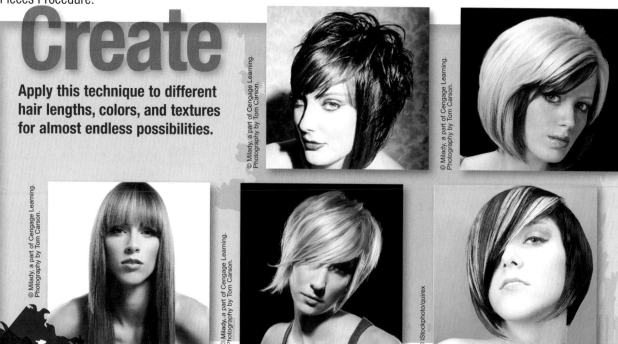

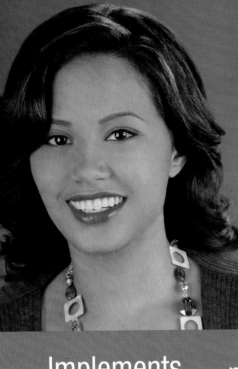

Accent Pieces— Baliage

Implements and Materials

You will need all of the following implements, materials, and supplies:

- **Towels**
- **Haircolor**
- **Lightener**
- **Developer**
- **Chemical cape**
- **Gloves**
- **Clips**
- **Comb**
- **Applicator bottle**
- **Bowl and brush**
- **Timer**
- **Client service record card**
- **Color chart**
- **Tail Comb**

Overview

The word baliage means "to paint." Whenever you want to add subtle highlights to make the top surface of the hair sparkle this is an easy, fun way to do so. The product you will use here is a powdered lightener.

Procedure

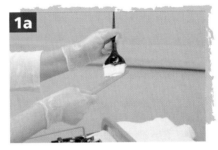

1a Put on gloves and mix lightener. Apply the powdered lightener to a styling comb, tail comb, or color brush.

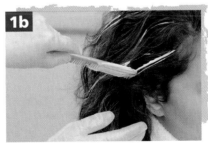

1b Lightly paint the product down the strand.

Formula: Lightener—an off-the-scalp lightener was used to lighten the hair. This product was mixed to the desired consistency with the manufacture dedicated 30-volume developer.

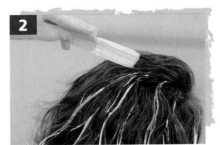

2 Work downward diagonally around the entire head.

Accent Pieces—Baliage continued

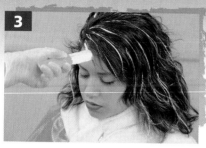

3 Once the baliage technique is completed, let it process for 10 to 15 minutes. Rinse and apply a color-enhancement formula over the highlighted hair if desired.*

* Depending on manufacturers recommendations, rinse or shampoo color product from the hair. Condition and finish as desired.

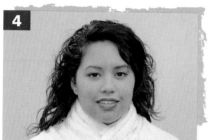

4 Before Dimensional Haircolor Services: Accent Pieces—Baliage Procedure.

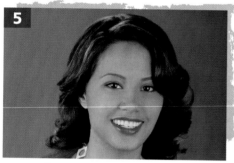

5 After Dimensional Haircolor Services: Accent Pieces—Baliage Procedure. Haircolor highlights strategically placed are a dramatic yet quick and practical addition.

Create

Apply this technique to different hair lengths, colors, and textures for almost endless possibilities.

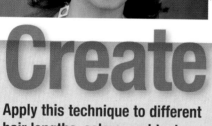
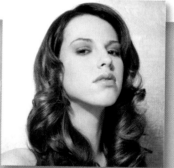
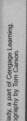
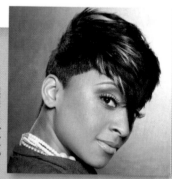
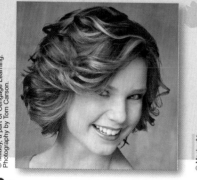
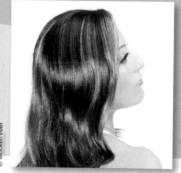
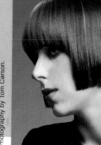
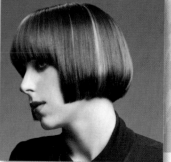

PART 6 Haircolor Challenges

Most haircolor challenges stem from a haircolor situation that has gone wrong. Over-highlighting hair that results in a very over-lightened blond look or haircolor that has been pulled through the ends over and over again resulting in very dark ends with a lighter regrowth area are two situations that can require correction. Sometimes the tone of a haircolor can be off or unattractive because of the formula applied or because the hair may have been overly porous and consequently processed off-tone. There are many variables that affect the haircolor result.

It is important to review the *Colorist Code of Conduct* to understand the steps that must be taken prior to a haircolor service. Here, we'll take a look at some very common haircolor situations that can be challenging to a colorist.

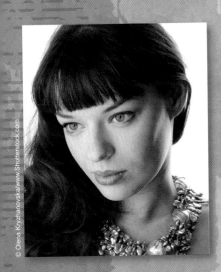

© Olena Kryzhanovska/www.Shutterstock.com

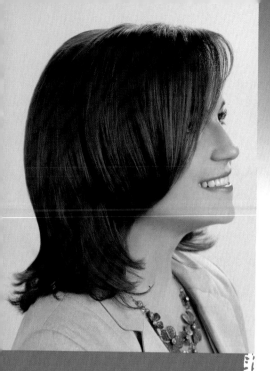

Challenge 1: Tinting Back Very Pale Blond to a Lighter Brown Shade

Implements and Materials

You will need all of the following implements, materials, and supplies:

- Towels
- Haircolor
- Lightener
- Developer
- Chemical cape
- Gloves
- Clips
- Comb
- Applicator bottle
- Bowl and brush
- Timer
- Client service record card
- Color chart
- Any special supplies needed to complete the procedure

Overview

One of the most important elements of haircoloring is knowing what you need to add to a color or what you need to remove from a color to create the best result. When a client come in and tells you that she wants to go back to her natural color…beware.

Think about this: They probably haven't seen their natural color in a long time. This is why softening the scalp area with a permanent color (Formula 1) for 15 minutes is a good idea. It will lighten the natural level slightly and make it easier to take it to a deeper shade.

Next, you will want to add back some warmth to the shaft and ends while the regrowth area is processing. This formula will be a demipermanent color (Formula 2) of warm tones to build back the missing warmth in the hair. Once the two formulas are on the different parts of the head, the color needs to process for up to 20 minutes. The hair will be rinsed and toweled dry.

A final glaze with a demipermanent color (Formula 3) will be applied to balance the entire color to finish it.

Procedure

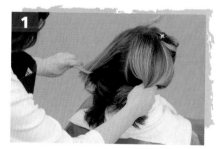

1 Section the hair into four sections. Apply protective cream to the hairline and ears.

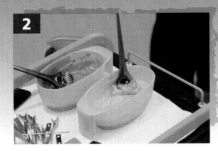

2 Put on gloves and mix Formula 1 and Formula 2 to create a permanent and demipermanent formula and set aside.

On our model we used the following formula:

- Formula 1—3parts 6N permanent haircolor with 3 parts 20-volume developer on regrowth area to soften the natural hair color.
- Formula 2—3 parts 6N demipermanent haircolor + 1 part warm tones (for example 6G, 6RO, to balance and fill lightened pieces) + equal portions demipermanent color developer.
- Formula 3—4 parts 5N demipermanent haircolor + 4 parts demipermanent haircolor developer.

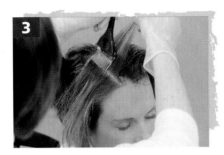

3 Outline all four sections with the permanent color product first. Then, beginning on the left front side, apply the permanent haircolor formula to the root area quickly. Continue applying the color to the other sections in the same manner.

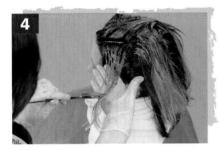

4 Immediately after finishing with the root application, begin applying the demipermanent color formula from the shaft to the ends in all four sections.

5 Set a timer for 20 minutes.

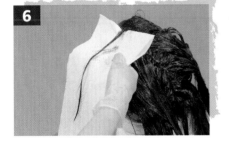

6 Strand test the color to see if they are similar and rinse with warm water.

Challenge 1: Tinting Back Very Pale Blond to a Lighter Brown Shade continued

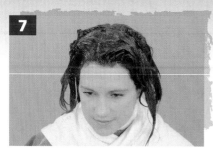

7 Towel-dry until hair is damp. Apply a final formula of a demipermanent color to the midshaft first. Apply from left front section, then move to the right front, left back, and right back. Once completed, apply from the scalp area to the ends on both sides of the strand. This final application will marry the finished color together. Set timer for 15 minutes.

8 Shampoo, condition, and style.

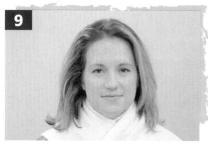

9 Before Tinting Back Very Pale Blond to a Lighter Brown Shade Procedure.

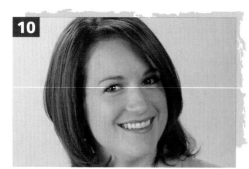

10 After Tinting Back Very Pale Blond to a Lighter Brown Shade Procedure. This technique can be used to take a light blond back to a brunette by altering the formulas. See the next procedure.

Create

Apply this technique to different hair lengths, colors, and textures for almost endless possibilities.

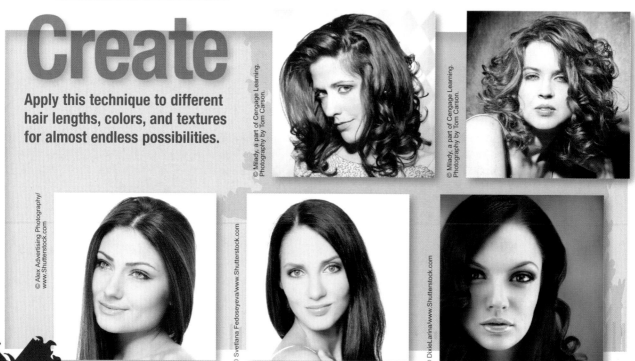

Part 1: Haircoloring

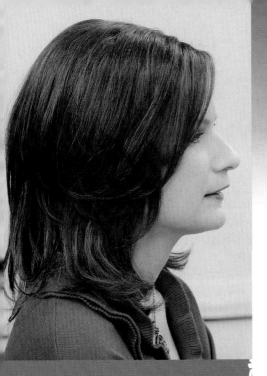

Challenge 2: Tinting Back Very Pale Blond Highlights to a Brown Shade

Implements and Materials

You will need all of the following implements, materials, and supplies:

- **Towels**
- **Haircolor**
- **Lightener**
- **Developer**
- **Chemical cape**
- **Gloves**
- **Clips**
- **Comb**
- **Applicator bottle**
- **Bowl and brush**
- **Timer**
- **Client service record card**
- **Color chart**
- **Any special supplies needed to complete the procedure**

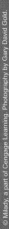
© Milady, a part of Cengage Learning. Photography by Gary David Gold.

Overview

In this tinting-back variation, you will be tinting back very pale blond hair to a lighter brown.

Tinting back is a process that requires the technician to apply permanent and demipermanent formulas to the scalp area and hair ends to add warmth and create a balance of color throughout the hair.

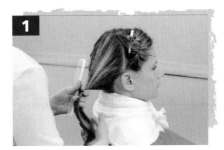

1 Part the hair into four sections. Apply protective cream to the hairline and ears.

2 Put on gloves and mix Formula 1 and Formula 2 and set aside.

On our model we used the following formula:

- Formula 1—3 parts 4N permanent haircolor with 3 parts 20-volume developer on regrowth area.
- Formula 2—1½ parts 4N demipermanent haircolor + ½ part warm tones (for example 6G, 6RO, to balance and fill lightened pieces) + equal portions demipermanent color developer.
- Formula 3—4 parts 4N demipermanent haircolor + 4 parts demipermanent haircolor developer.

Challenge 2: Tinting Back Very Pale Blond Highlights to a Brown Shade continued

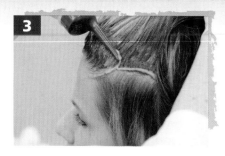

3 Outline all four sections with the permanent color product first. Then, beginning on the left front side, apply the permanent haircolor formula to the root area quickly. Continue applying the color to the other sections in the same manner.

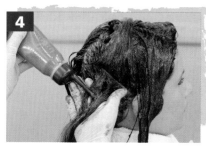

4 Immediately after finishing with the root application, begin applying the demipermanent color formula from the shaft to the ends in all four sections.

5 Set timer for 20 minutes.

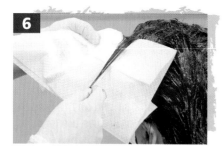

6 Strand test the color to see if they are similar and rinse with warm water.

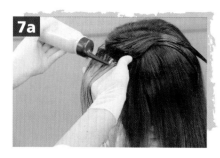

7a Towel-dry until hair is damp. Apply a final formula of a demipermanent color and begin applying from the ends up to the scalp area.

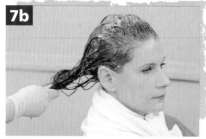

7b This final demipermanent glaze will marry the two shades of color together.

7c Set timer for 15 minutes.

8 Shampoo, condition, and style.

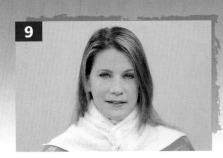

9 Before Tinting Back Very Pale Blond Highlights to a Brown Shade Procedure.

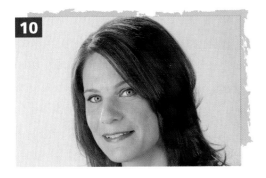

10 After Tinting Back Very Pale Blond Highlights to a Brown Shade Procedure.

Create

Apply this technique to different hair lengths, colors, and textures for almost endless possibilities.

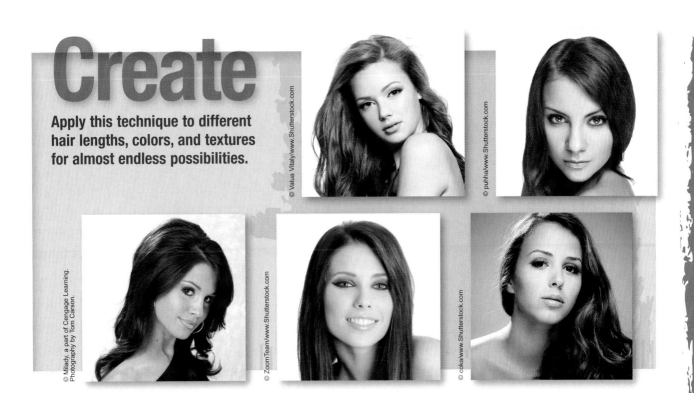

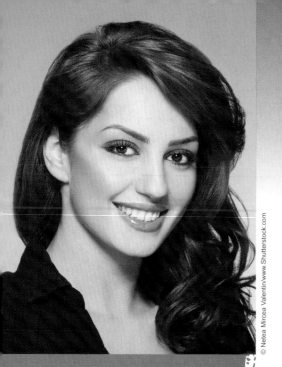

Challenge 3: Neutralizing Unwanted Ash Tones

Implements and Materials

You will need all of the following implements, materials, and supplies:

- **Towels**
- **Haircolor**
- **Lightener**
- **Developer**
- **Chemical cape**
- **Gloves**
- **Clips**
- **Comb**
- **Applicator bottle**
- **Bowl and brush**
- **Timer**
- **Client service record card**
- **Color chart**
- **Any special supplies needed to complete the procedure**

Overview

Unwanted tones can be present in a color for many reasons. Incorrect formulas with the wrong tones can sometimes process bright, drab, or just off-tone. Sometimes gray or white hair will process brighter, which can be neutralized easily. One trick to remember when neutralizing unwanted tones is to recall which color is opposite the unwanted tone on the color wheel.

Procedure

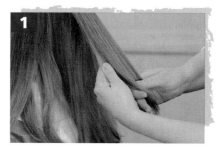

1 Determine unwanted tone in the hair. In this case, the unwanted tone is an ash or green tone. Comb through the hair and part into four sections. Apply protective cream to the hairline and ears.

2 Mix the proper color formula, keeping in mind that orange will neutralize an ash tone.

On our model we used the following formula:
- Formula 1—3 parts 6N permanent haircolor with 3 parts 20-volume developer on regrowth area.
- Formula 2—1½ parts 6N demipermanent haircolor + ½ part warm tones (for example 6G, 6RO, to balance and fill lightened pieces) + equal portions demipermanent color developer.

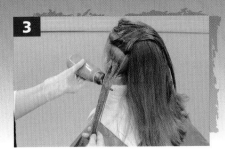

3 Apply the formula to the parts of the hair that need to be neutralized. In this case, you will apply color from the midshaft to the ends all around the head.

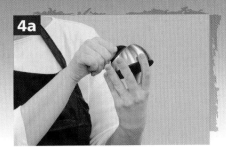

4a Once color is applied to all areas, set a timer.

4b Check every 5 minutes until the desired results are achieved.

4c Shampoo, condition, and style.

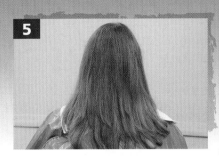

5 Before Neutralizing Unwanted Ash Tones Procedure.

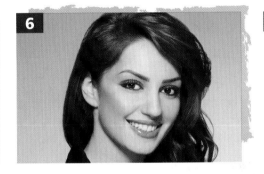

6 After Neutralizing Unwanted Ash Tones Procedure.

Create

Apply this technique to different hair lengths, colors, and textures for almost endless possibilities.

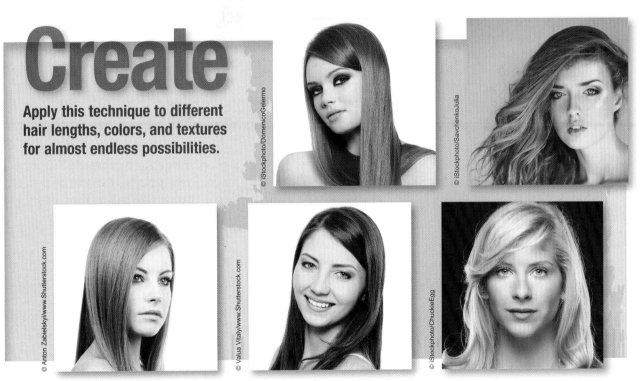

Part 1: Haircoloring

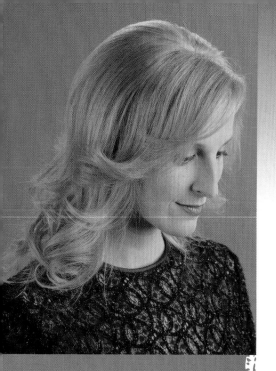

Challenge 4: Neutralizing Unwanted Brassy Tones

Implements and Materials

You will need all of the following implements, materials, and supplies:

- **Towels**
- **Haircolor**
- **Lightener**
- **Developer**
- **Chemical cape**
- **Gloves**
- **Clips**
- **Comb**
- **Applicator bottle**
- **Bowl and brush**
- **Timer**
- **Client service record card**
- **Color chart**
- **Any special supplies needed to complete the procedure**

Overview

If hair is brassy or orange, the color opposite it on the color wheel is blue—which means a cool-based color should correct the brassy tone. If hair is very warm or yellow, the opposite of it on the color wheel is violet.

If you are faced with these haircolor situations, here are some simple rules to help you create the haircolor result you want to achieve.

Procedure

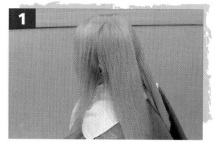

1 Determine unwanted tone in the hair. In this case, the unwanted tone is a brassy-orange and it is present throughout the strand. Comb through the hair and part into four sections.

2 Now, put on gloves and mix the proper formula, keeping in mind that blue is the opposite color of orange.

On our model we used the following formula:
- Formula 1—1½ parts 12N permanent haircolor with 3 parts 40-volume developer on regrowth area.
- Formula 2—3 parts 8N demipermanent haircolor + equal portions demipermanent color developer.

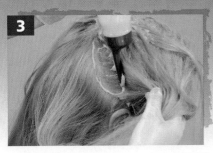

3 Outline each section and apply the color product to the root area of all four sections. Once the color product has been applied to the root area, return to the section you started with and apply the color to the rest of the hair strand.

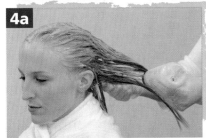

4a Work the color through to the ends. Be sure the hair is completely saturated with color. When you have finished applying the color, work it through the hair.

4b Once color is applied to all areas, set a timer and check every 5 minutes until the desired results are achieved.

4c Shampoo, condition, and style.

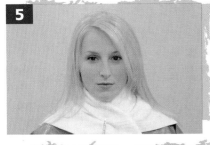

5 Before Neutralizing Unwanted Brassy Tones Procedure.

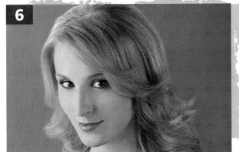

6 After Neutralizing Unwanted Brassy Tones Procedure.

Create

Apply this technique to different hair lengths, colors, and textures for almost endless possibilities.

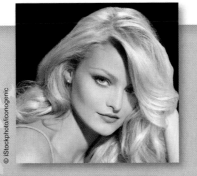
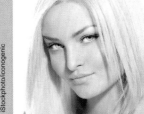

© iStockphoto/iconogenic

© iStockphoto/iconogenic

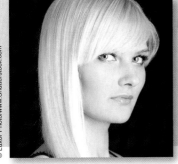
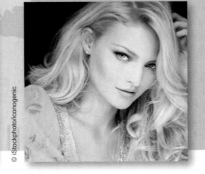
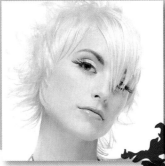

© Luxor Photo/www.Shutterstock.com

© iStockphoto/iconogenic

© iStockphoto/Lercha&Johnson

Part 1: Haircoloring

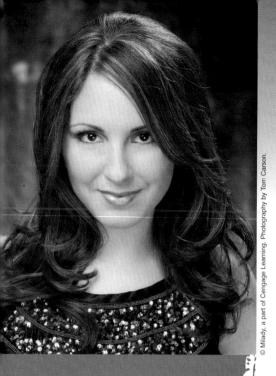

Challenge 5: Removing Dark Color from the Ends

Implements and Materials

You will need all of the following implements, materials, and supplies:

- Towels
- Haircolor
- Color Remover
- Developer
- Chemical cape
- Gloves
- Clips
- Comb
- Applicator bottle
- Bowl and brush
- Timer
- Client service record card
- Color chart
- Any special supplies needed to complete the procedure

Overview

Haircolor that builds up on the ends and creates discoloration can result from many things. Sometimes, bringing color down through the ends repeatedly after it is applied to the regrowth area can cause unnecessary and unwanted depth. Overly porous hair can grab color on the ends, resulting in deeper color on the ends than on the rest of the strand.

Whatever created the situations above, it can usually be reversed.

Procedure

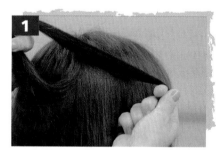

1 Determine the area that has dark color and must be lightened.

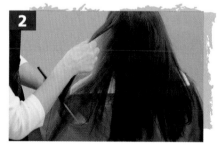

2 Examine the rest of the hair to see if there is anything that has to be adjusted. If a color has to be placed at the regrowth, formulate the color and apply.

3 Mix a color remover (following the manufacturer's directions).

On our model we used the following formula:
1 scoop on-the-scalp lightener + 1 part 20-volume developer + 3 pumps shampoo.

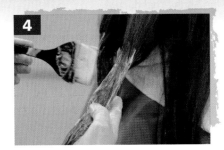

4 Apply the color remover to the dark pieces quickly. Completely saturate these sections. Work it through with your hands.

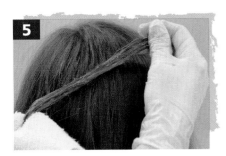

5 Check the hair to see when it starts lifting. Remember, you want the hair to get as close to the desired color as possible.

6 Once you have achieved the desired lift, rinse the hair. It will appear to be orange or very brassy. At this time, you will be rinsing the color from the regrowth area as well. (Both the application of color to the regrowth and the color remover will take around 30 minutes.)

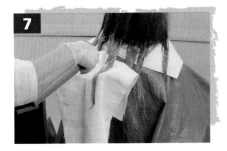

7 Determine the formula to neutralize the orange tones and use a demipermanent color if desired. (Step not required on model shown.)

8a Apply the color formula, working from the ends up, on the orange color. Set a timer. Check the color every 5 minutes until desired color is reached.

8b Shampoo, condition, and style.

Challenge 5: Removing Dark Color from the Ends continued

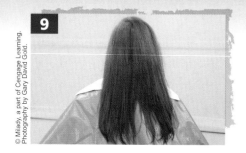

9 Before Removing Dark Color from the Ends Procedure.

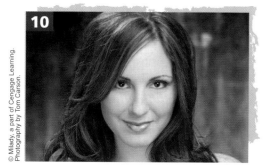

10 After Removing Dark Color from the Ends Procedure.

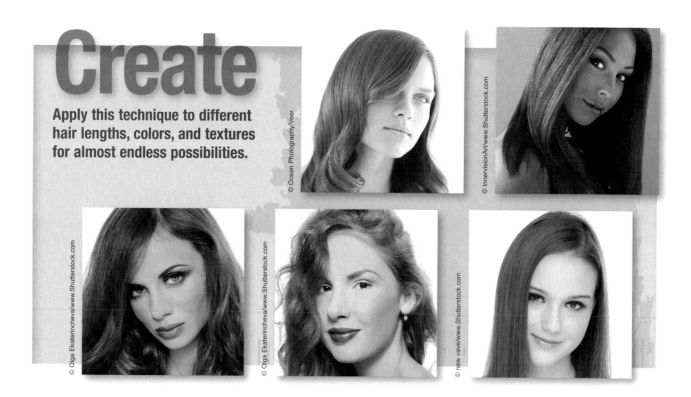

Create

Apply this technique to different hair lengths, colors, and textures for almost endless possibilities.

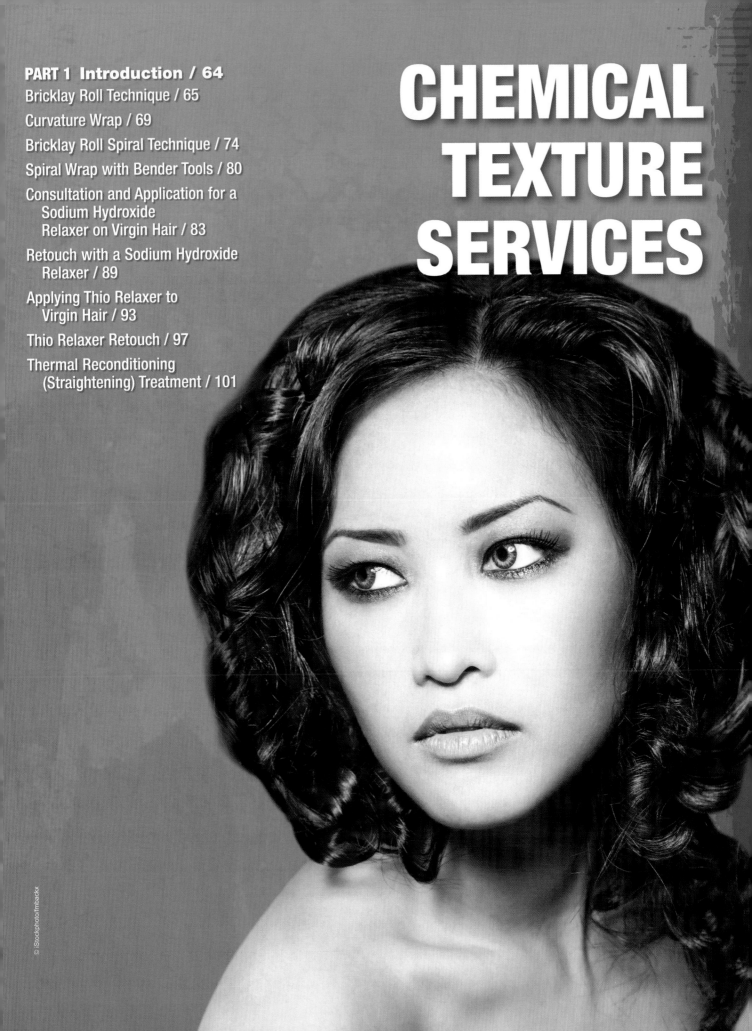

CHEMICAL TEXTURE SERVICES

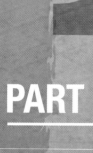

PART 1

Introduction

Clients today want instant gratification with their hairstyles. This includes the results of their texture services—a client wants to comb through or run her fingers through her hair and have it fall into place effortlessly.

Before any texture service, always perform a complete hair analysis. The hair's condition, texture, wave pattern, strength, and porosity will guide your selection of a perming or relaxing product, type and size of perm rod, and wrapping technique. Until you gain experience, use a double end paper wrap, which allows greater control.

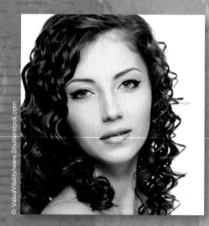

© ValuaVitality/www.Shutterstock.com

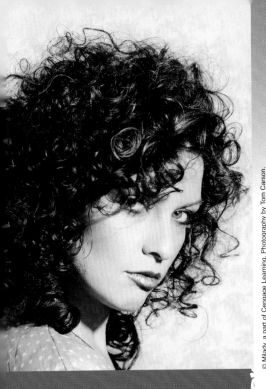

Bricklay Roll Technique

Implements and Materials

You will need all of the following implements, materials, and supplies:

- **Clarifying shampoo (optional)**
- **Applicator bottles**
- **Conditioner (optional)**
- **Cotton coil or rope**
- **Disposable gloves**
- **End papers**
- **Neutralizer**
- **Neutralizing bib**
- **Perm rods**
- **Perm solution**
- **Plastic clips for sectioning**
- **Plastic tail comb**
- **Pre-neutralizing conditioner (optional)**
- **Protective barrier cream**
- **Roller picks**
- **Chemical cape**
- **Spray bottle**
- **Styling comb**
- **Timer**
- **Towels**

Overview

In this section, you will explore using the bricklay permanent wrap technique to set the entire head. This setting pattern will be one of the most frequently used in the salon. The flow of movement in the finished result looks natural and can be easily maintained by your client. Hair flows with no discernible splits between rows. The bricklay permanent wrap technique will expand and enhance voluminous movement and dimension. The tool diameters used here will create a firm, resilient curl pattern.

The backswept direction off the face opens up and keeps hair from falling in the face. It moves hair back and up against the natural fall of gravity, creating desirable volume. The setting pattern involves beginning at the front forehead area with the first tool placed. This serves as the starting point for all subsequent partings through the top and sides to parallel each other. At the crown, horizontal partings are taken that continue down to the nape.

The finished results can be varied by using zigzag partings to avoid splits or by alternating rod sizes to create a mix of larger and smaller curls. You can also use different base controls to alter the results, or direct all the hair around the front hairline toward the face. Once you have mastered the bricklay permanent wrap technique, experiment with these variations to enhance your creativity and customize the look for your client.

Technical Drawing

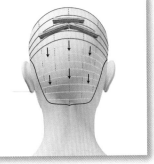

Bricklay Roll Technique continued

Procedure

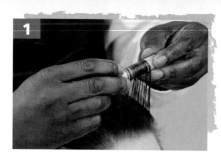

1 Begin wrapping at the front hairline area by parting a base area that is the length and width of the longer rod you are using. At the hairline, comb and distribute the hair 90 degrees above the center of the base area. Apply a double end paper wrap. Roll from the ends to the base, and position the rod half off base to minimize tension at the hairline. On base wrapping could cause breakage in this area.

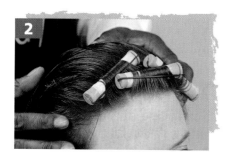

2 In the row directly behind your first rod, take base partings that allow for two midlength rods to be offset from the center of the first rod. Partings that are not at the fragile hairline should be wrapped at 45 degrees above the center of the base and positioned on base for maximum volume.

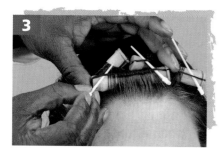

3 Insert picks underneath the bands to alleviate pressure on the hair.

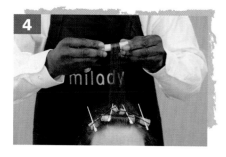

4 Before you set the next row, study the area to be wrapped. Adjust the rod length as needed to accommodate this area. Now, begin the next row by positioning a rod at the center of the spot where the two rods met in the previous row.

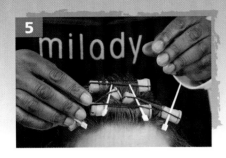

5 The pattern you see here is the one you will use to wrap the entire head. Work quickly, precisely, and methodically.

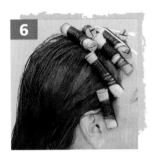

6 Continue to part rows that radiate around the curve of the head, extending around and down toward the side hairline area. Maintain precision partings, distribution, and rolling of hair strands to create the bricklay pattern. Secure the rods and insert picks, either as you go or when you have finished wrapping.

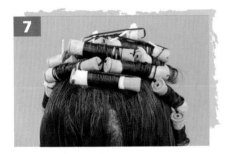

7 At the crown area of the head, instead of curving rows around the front hairline, take rows that work around the back of the head in a horizontal fashion. Continue with the bricklay pattern. As you work from row to row, adjust the length of the rod to fit into the area you are working on.

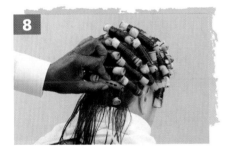

8 When you reach the occipital area, you may want to change to a smaller rod to create more curl definition and support. When lengths become quite short, change your end paper technique. Fold a single end paper in half and bookend wrap to control and smooth the ends.

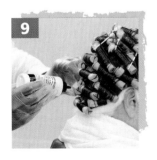

9 As you move toward the perimeter or nape, complete the wrap using a one-diameter base size with the rod positioned half off base. Apply a barrier cream around the hairline and ears, and wrap a cotton coil around the entire hairline. Put gloves on both hands. Now, saturate both sides of each rod with the perm solution. Process according to manufacturer's directions and take a test curl. When processing is completed, rinse for at least 5 minutes, then blot thoroughly before neutralizing.

Bricklay Roll Technique continued

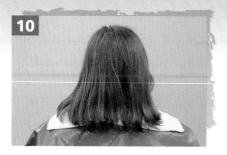

10 Before Bricklay Roll Technique Procedure service.

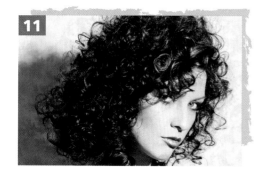

11 After Bricklay Roll Texture Procedure service.

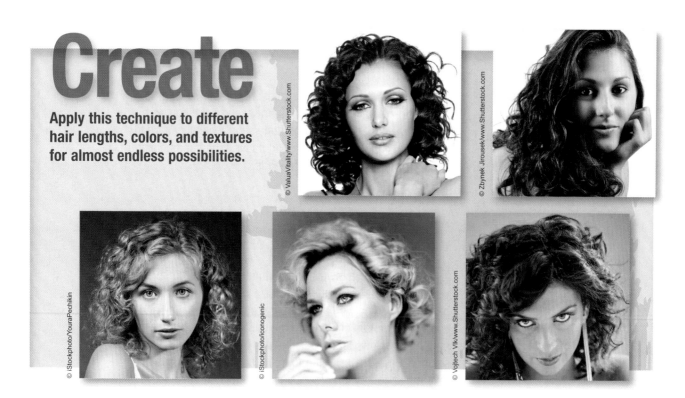

Create

Apply this technique to different hair lengths, colors, and textures for almost endless possibilities.

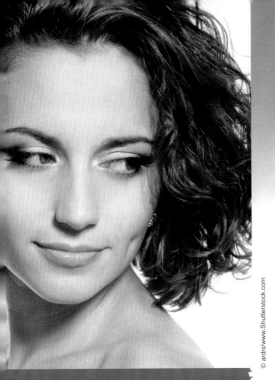
© ardni/www.Shutterstock.com

Curvature Wrap

Implements and Materials

You will need all of the following implements, materials, and supplies:

- **Clarifying shampoo (optional)**
- **Applicator bottles**
- **Conditioner (optional)**
- **Cotton coil or rope**
- **Disposable gloves**
- **End papers**
- **Neutralizer**
- **Neutralizing bib**
- **Perm rods**
- **Perm solution**
- **Plastic clips for sectioning**
- **Plastic tail comb**
- **Pre-neutralizing conditioner (optional)**
- **Protective barrier cream**
- **Roller picks**
- **Chemical cape**
- **Spray bottle**
- **Styling comb**
- **Timer**
- **Towels**

Overview

In this wrap, the panels used throughout the head have a directional emphasis to them—they contour to the curves of the head. This curvature panel setting creates a seamless flow of texture throughout the central region of the head, from the front hairline to the nape, which complements the Heavily Layered Haircut. The flow of hair is very natural, as well as extremely manageable for the client.

Essentially, curvature panel wrapping takes into account the desired style lines and how the client will wear her hair, making styling easier for her. For this layered haircut, rod sizes alternate within the panels. The rods are rolled for volume up to the perimeter, where an indentation application creates a more closely contoured effect. In addition, the area framing the face is set within a curvature motion. Contrast this to block setting, in which lines are rigidly set in a downward directional throughout the exterior of the set.

The movement created throughout the interior allows for the hair to blend beautifully from the front forehead area to the back.

Technical Drawing

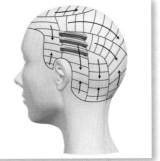
© Milady, a part of Cengage Learning

Curvature Wrap continued
Procedure

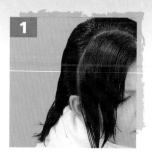

1 Begin by sectioning the curvature panels throughout the entire head. Comb the hair in the direction that it will move, then section individual panels to match the length of the chosen rod. Begin this procedure at the front hairline area off of the side part area.

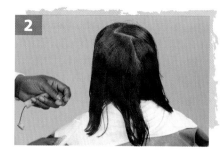

2 Alternate from side to side, as you section the panels and clip them out of the way. Here is the finished sectioning pattern from the back.

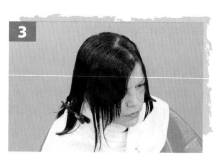

3 Pre-sectioning of the curvature panels you will use to roll this texture wrap will allow you to wrap neatly and in clear directions—it will give you a road map or blueprint to follow.

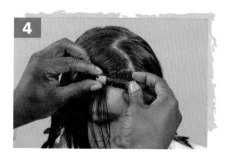

4 Begin the curvature wrapping at the front hairline area, next to the side parting. Part a one-diameter base size and roll the rod to the on base position. If potential breakage is a concern, use a 90-degee angle for half off base wrapping in the fragile hairline area.

5 Stabilize your rods with picks as needed while you roll.

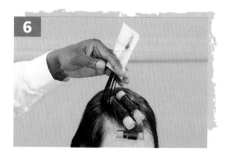

6 As you work through the panel, continue parting base sections that are expanded around the outside area of the panel, the area farthest away from the face. Keep in mind that the base areas should always be no larger than the diameter of the rod. When you reach the crest area working over the curve of the head, distribute the hair straight out from the base area to position the rod half off base.

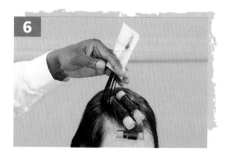

© Milady, a part of Cengage Learning. Photography by Gary David Gold.

Part 2: Chemical Texture Services

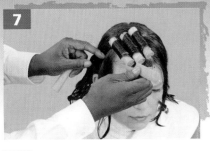

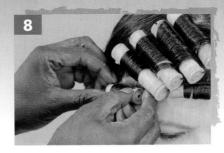

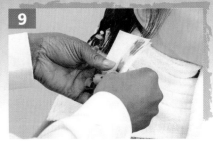

7   Note how the base is being parted out of the panel so as not to disturb the surrounding hair. Lift it out and around in a curve.

8   Use a smaller diameter rod and alternate rod diameters as you work toward the perimeter.

9   When you reach the last rod to be rolled, comb the hair flat at the base and position the rod in preparation for rolling up and away.

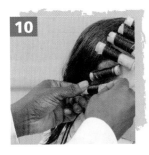

10   Roll the rod up and toward the base, while keeping the base area flat. Roll perimeter lengths in the indentation technique. This will maintain closely contoured movement within this area.

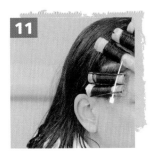

11   Because of the flat base you get with an upward-rolled rod, insert the pick in an upward direction.

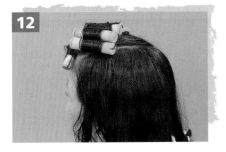

12   Move to the other side of the head, and set the panel around the hairline on the lighter side of the part, using the same technique. Here, the first few rods are placed.

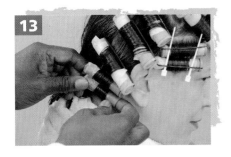

13   Next, move to the panel behind and adjacent to the first one you set. Roll rods with an on base rod control throughout the top area of the head; change to a half off base control toward the exterior, until you reach the perimeter area. Set the last two rods in each panel in the indentation technique to accentuate the effect.

Curvature Wrap continued

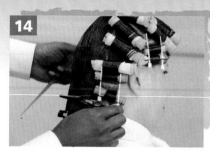

14 Add a pick after rolling; the upward-directed rod requires support.

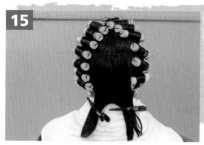

15 Return to the panel on the opposite side of the head and roll for volume, using the same technique and alternating rod sizes within the panel. Here is the back of the head with two panels left to roll.

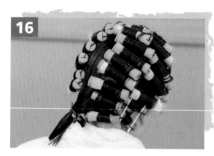

16 Roll all rods for volume in this panel until you reach the perimeter area, where you should roll the rods upward for indentation.

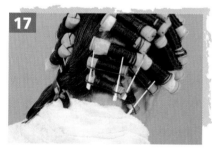

17 Insert picks to secure the rods and ease any band tension on the hair.

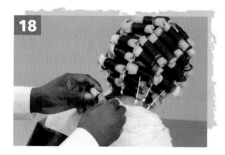

18 Complete the last panel. Note that the directional movement within this panel should remain consistent with the pattern you have already established. The directional movement throughout the back flows around and contours to the perimeter hairline area.

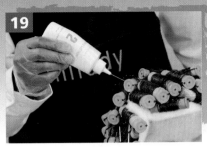

19 Apply a barrier cream around the hairline and ears, and wrap a cotton coil around the entire hairline. Put gloves on both hands. Then saturate both sides of each rod with the perm solution. Process according to manufacturer's directions, and take a test curl. When processing is completed, rinse for at least 5 minutes, then blot thoroughly before neutralizing.

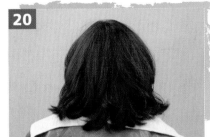

20 Before Curvature Wrap Procedure service.

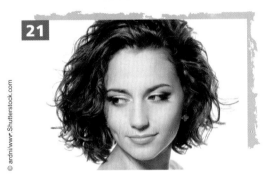

21 After Curvature Wrap Procedure service. In the finished look, the hair has been diffused dry—this is the most representative finish of the wave set. Note the flicked-out areas around the perimeter, which combine and harmonize with the mix of voluminous texture throughout the interior.

Create

Apply this technique to different hair lengths, colors, and textures for almost endless possibilities.

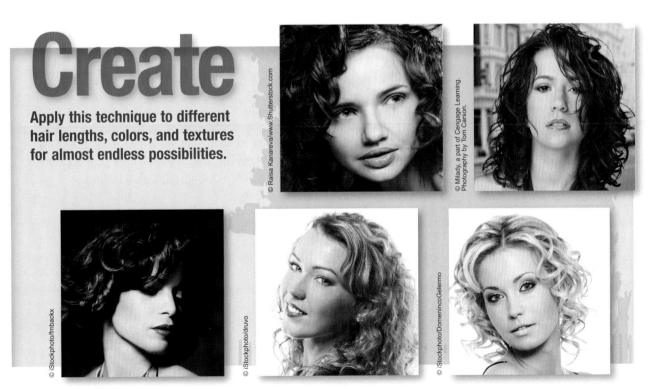

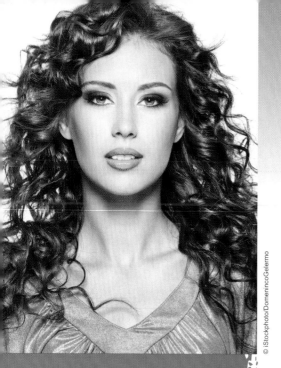

Implements and Materials

You will need all of the following implements, materials, and supplies:

- **Clarifying shampoo (optional)**
- **Applicator bottles**
- **Conditioner (optional)**
- **Cotton coil or rope**
- **Disposable gloves**
- **End papers**
- **Neutralizer**
- **Neutralizing bib**
- **Perm rods**
- **Perm solution**
- **Plastic clips for sectioning**
- **Plastic tail comb**
- **Pre-neutralizing conditioner (optional)**
- **Protective barrier cream**
- **Roller picks**
- **Chemical cape**
- **Spray bottle**
- **Styling comb**
- **Timer**
- **Towels**

Bricklay Roll Spiral Technique

Overview

The bricklay pattern is a classic technique for arranging or setting the tools in position for waving. It creates a smooth flow of movement because base partings are offset from row to row. In this design, we transform the shoulder-length Horizontal Blunt Haircut to create luxurious wave patterns, movement, and dimension. The nape area is rolled horizontally, using a bricklay pattern. This creates expansion and undulation. The rest of the hair is spiral wrapped with larger tools to create elongated ringlets.

The rolling and spiraling techniques are fundamental for creating a wide variety of textural effects. The techniques remain the same whether the pattern of application is within direction, curvature, or straight movements.

The rolling technique, sometimes called *croquignole wrapping*, involves rotating the tool to wrap the hair evenly around it (similar to the way you would roll up a diploma or scroll). Distribute the hair evenly along the tool as you roll smoothly toward the base. This creates a strong undulation.

The spiraling technique involves winding a strand of hair along a tool from one end to the other. (Think of how the stripes on a barber pole appear to spiral around it.) This creates natural-looking, elongated texture.

Technical Drawing

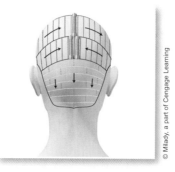

Part 2: Chemical Texture Services

Procedure

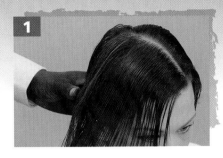

1 Begin the procedure by sectioning the hair using a side part, curving toward the center crown.

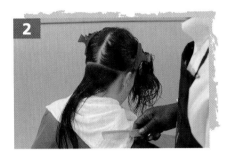

2 Start at the center crown and part down the center back vertically. To subdivide the nape area, part horizontally from the occipital area to the center back of the ear on both sides.

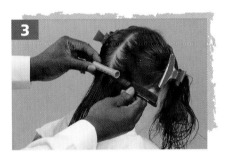

3 Begin at the top center area of the nape section by placing the rod and parting to the length and width of the rod (a one-diameter base size).

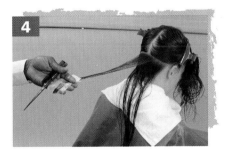

4 Comb the hair straight out from the base parting and place two end papers over the ends in preparation for rolling the hair smoothly.

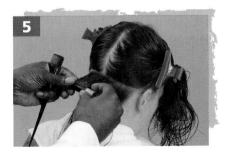

5 Position the rod at the ends and begin to roll the hair smoothly toward the base area, maintaining the hair position (straight out from the base) as you roll. When you reach the base area, secure the band and cap across the rod.

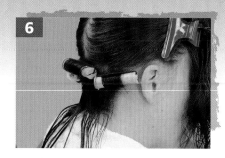

6 Continue to roll the hair lengths on either side of this center rod. Use the appropriate rod length and number of rods needed to complete this row.

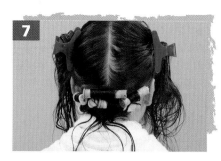

7 Offset the rod positioning in the next row from the center top rod. This will ensure no hair splits between rows. Adjust rod length as needed to adapt for your client's head size, hairline, etc.

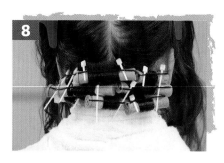

8 Complete the bricklay rolling technique in the nape area. Position picks through the bands. Turn the band toward the top of the rod before inserting the pick. The completed nape area indicates a bricklay pattern with horizontally rolled rods.

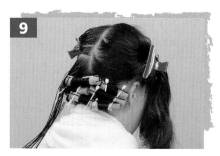

9 Part 1-inch (2.5 cm) wide subsections, for spiraling the hair onto rods vertically from center back to the front hairline. The 1-inch (2.5 cm) width can vary, depending on the amount of base lift desired.

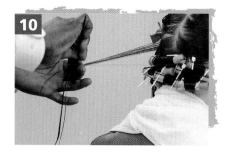

10 Part vertical base sections that are approximately the width of the rod. Comb the lengths diagonally outward from the base area in preparation for spiraling the hair.

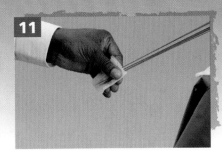

11 Fold the end paper in a bookend style over the ends.

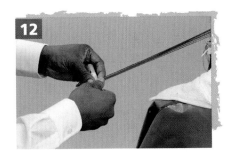

12 Place the end of the rod at the ends of the hair and roll at least one and a half revolutions to secure the ends.

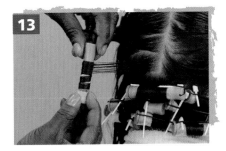

13 With the ends secure, spiral the hair onto the rod. Secure the rod when you reach the base area.

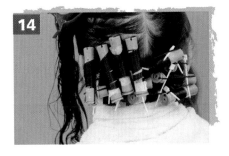

14 Continue to use this method of spiraling lengths onto the rod as you move toward the side front hairline area. Maintain consistent hair sections as you spiral wrap the hair. Wrap so that the open ends are toward the face. Then repeat the procedure on the opposite side of this section.

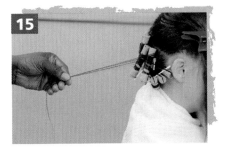

15 As you work upward and around the head, continue to divide the hair into the 1-inch (2.5 cm) subsections as seen here for the last rod of the first vertically wrapped section.

Bricklay Roll Spiral Technique continued

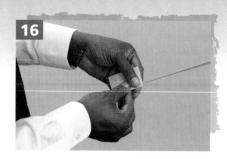

16 Be aware of the distribution from the curve of the head. Hold the hair diagonally outward before positioning the end paper and spiraling.

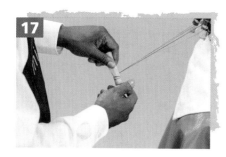

17 Secure the ends of the hair (one and a half to two revolutions) at one end of the rod, and then proceed to spiral lengths along the rod.

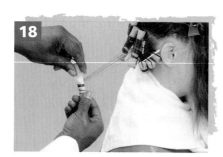

18 Maintain a slight diagonal on the rod as you spiral toward the base, before fastening to secure. Continue to work upward and around the head, subdividing sections until the wrap is completed.

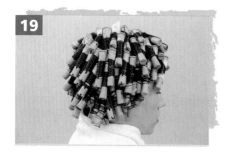

19 In the finished wrap, each row overlaps the previous sections. When wrapping is completed, apply a barrier cream around the hairline and ears and wrap a cotton coil around the entire hairline. Put gloves on both hands. Next, saturate both sides of each rod with the perm solution. Process according to manufacturer's directions and take a test curl. When processing is completed, rinse for at least 5 minutes, then blot thoroughly before neutralizing.

© Milady, a part of Cengage Learning. Photography by Gary David Gold.

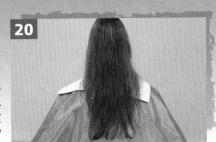

20 Before Bricklay Roll Spiral Technique Procedure service.

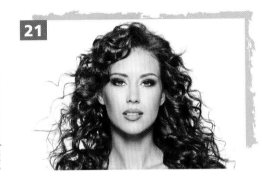

21 After Bricklay Roll Spiral Technique Procedure service. The finished look shows luxurious spirals with support underneath. This technique may be adapted to create a wide variety of effects. The finished texture creates dimension and adds dynamic movement to the Blunt Haircut.

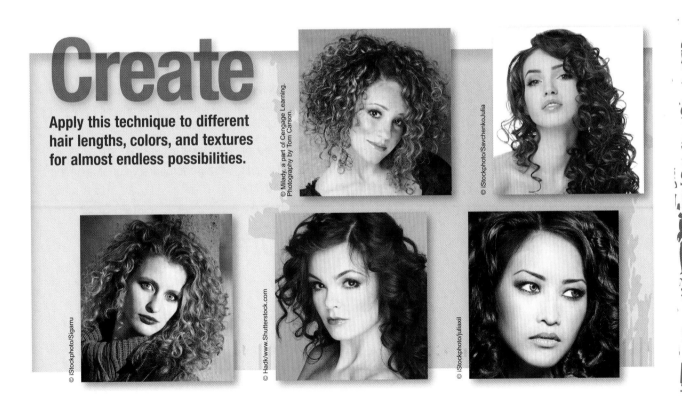

Create

Apply this technique to different hair lengths, colors, and textures for almost endless possibilities.

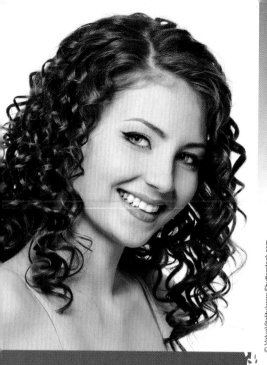

© ValuaVitality/www.Shutterstock.com

Spiral Wrap with Bender Tools

Implements and Materials

You will need all of the following implements, materials, and supplies:

- **Clarifying shampoo (optional)**
- **Applicator bottles**
- **Conditioner (optional)**
- **Cotton coil or rope**
- **Disposable gloves**
- **End papers**
- **Neutralizer**
- **Neutralizing bib**
- **Bender tools (varying sizes)**
- **Perm solution**
- **Plastic clips for sectioning**
- **Plastic tail comb**
- **Pre-neutralizing conditioner (optional)**
- **Protective barrier cream**
- **Roller picks**
- **Chemical cape**
- **Spray bottle**
- **Styling comb**
- **Timer**
- **Towels**

Overview

In this procedure, the spiral technique is used on the Light Layers Haircut to create enhanced volume throughout its shape. This shows the versatility of the spiral technique—which can be adapted to all lengths of hair. In this wrapping technique, you will use soft bender rods to spiral the hair lengths. These rods come in a variety of diameters and lengths.

Adjust your choices according to the length of hair and the desired results. Here, a progression of diameters is used—smaller throughout the nape area, progressing to larger throughout the crest and top. You can also alternate wrapping directions for varied effects.

When working with longer hair, speed and efficiency are key. These same tools are frequently used in roller sets to create temporary curl. Mastering their use will only extend your artistry.

Technical Drawing

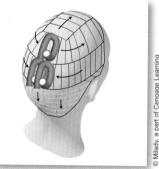

© Milady, a part of Cengage Learning

Procedure

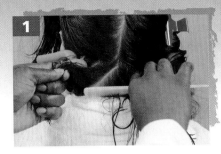

1 Begin at the nape with the smallest-sized tool you have selected. Working from the perimeter toward the center, take partings on a diagonal to create a directional influence in that section.

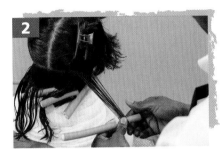

2 After completely wrapping the nape area, move up and wrap a second row above the first to complete wrapping all of the hair in the nape area.

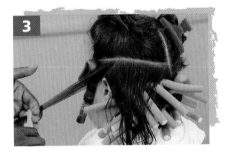

3 After completely wrapping the nape area, move to the sides and wrap the hair in the same manner, alternating directions within each row. This time, use larger-sized tools. This wrapping pattern follows the same progression throughout the head as the Bricklay Roll Spiral Technique.

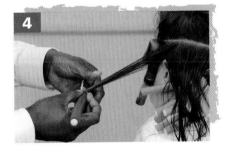

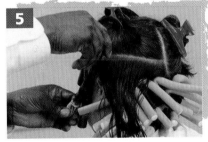

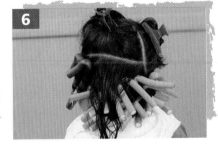

4 Always comb the hair lengths on a diagonal from the base area. Secure the ends of the hair at one end of the tool by revolving or rolling the ends one and a half to two turns around the tool.

5 Then begin spiraling the remaining lengths of hair toward the base area.

6 Secure the tool at the base area by turning its end in the opposite direction from how you spiraled the hair. Continue working around the head and up in this manner.

7 In the finished wrap, you can see the progression of the rod diameter sizes—smaller at the nape area and larger at the crest and top area of the head.

Spiral Wrap with Bender Tools continued

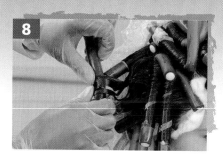

8 When wrapping is completed, put gloves on both hands and apply a barrier cream around the hairline and ears, then wrap a cotton coil around the entire hairline. Next, saturate both sides of each tool with the perm solution. Process according to manufacturer's directions and take a test curl. When processing is completed, rinse for at least 5 minutes, taking extra care to rinse all sides very well when using these tools. Blot thoroughly before neutralizing.

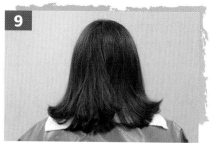

9 Before Spiral Wrap with Bender Tools Procedure service.

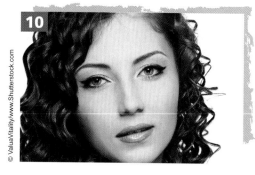

10 After Spiral Wrap with Bender Tools Procedure service. The finished style shows an undulating progression of textures. The spirals add liveliness and mobility to longer hair.

© ValuaVitality/www.Shutterstock.com

© Milady, a part of Cengage Learning. Photography by Gary David Gold.

Create

Apply this technique to different hair lengths, colors, and textures for almost endless possibilities.

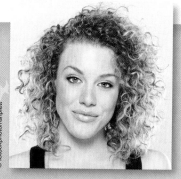

© iStockphoto/ranplett

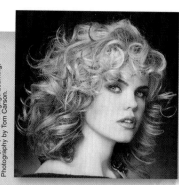

© Milady, a part of Cengage Learning. Photography by Tom Carson.

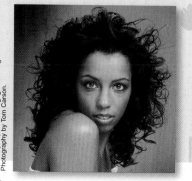

© Milady, a part of Cengage Learning. Photography by Tom Carson.

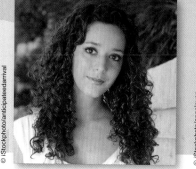

© iStockphoto/anticipateedarrival

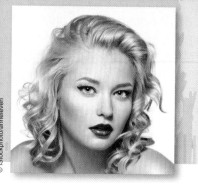

© iStockphoto/anneleven

82

Part 2: Chemical Texture Services

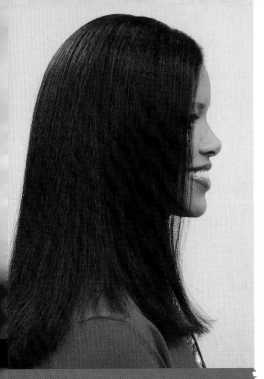

Consultation and Application for a Sodium Hydroxide Relaxer on Virgin Hair

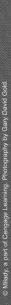

© Milady, a part of Cengage Learning. Photography by Gary David Gold.

Implements and Materials

You will need all of the following implements, materials, and supplies:

- Acid-balanced shampoo
- Bowl and applicator brush
- Conditioner
- Disposable gloves
- Hard rubber comb
- Hydroxide neutralizer
- Hydroxide relaxer
- Plastic clips
- Protective base cream
- Chemical cape
- Spray bottle
- Styling comb
- Timer
- Towels

Overview

Sodium Hydroxide is the most popular relaxing product for clients who have extremely curly hair, but it can also be used on slightly lesser degrees of curl. During a virgin relaxing service, the combination of the relaxer and a minimal amount of mechanical stress straightens the hair. The manipulation of the hair is the key to a successful service.

When performed properly, the processing technique will yield superb results. A complete hair and scalp analysis is required. Never proceed if the hair is damaged or the scalp has abrasions. Do not use a sodium hydroxide product on hair that has been exposed to professional lighteners or vice versa. (Many clients may call this "bleached" hair.) Also, never use a sodium hydroxide product on hair that has been exposed to a thio-based product.

The product's strength should be chosen according to the hair's condition, type, curl pattern, and exposure to previous chemical services. In general, a mild/gentle relaxer is appropriate for fine or tinted hair, medium/regular strength is appropriate for most medium-textured hair, and strong/super-strength formulations, which are not commonly used, are appropriate for very coarse, resistant hair.

Extremely curly hair tends to be porous and the more porous the hair, the faster it will process. The average processing time for a relaxing service is 13 to 15 minutes. Relaxers also come as regular or no-base. Unless you are using a no-base product, the entire scalp should be protected with a barrier cream. Always apply a protective cream around the client's entire hairline and follow manufacturer's instructions precisely.

The hair should be completely dry; do not shampoo the hair before relaxing. Always wear gloves. Your hands can become sensitized to the chemicals over a period of time, creating vulnerability for allergic reaction or contact dermatitis.

Consultation and Application for a Sodium Hydroxide Relaxer on Virgin Hair continued

The application should begin in the most resistant area—usually the back of the head. Use ½-inch (1.25 cm) partings and make certain the product is distributed evenly. Using a brush-and-bowl application and applying the relaxer to both sides of the parting are the best ways to ensure an even and efficient application.

Once the application is completed, the hair must be smoothed to add mechanical action to the process. Use minimal tension and press the partings with the back of a comb. Never comb through the hair with the comb's teeth. Once these smoothing/pressing steps have been completed, take a test strand and continue to do so every few minutes.

If your client also wants haircolor, color services can be performed 1 or 2 weeks after the relaxing service. Do not attempt same-day chemical services—even with a semipermanent color product—until you have mastered relaxing and thoroughly understand combined chemical services. Never highlight this hair with lightener.

Like all permanent relaxers, a sodium hydroxide relaxer affects the strands by permanently rearranging the basic structure of curly hair into a new, straightened form. For a successful service, begin with an understanding of the hair's current condition and texture while also considering the desired condition and texture. Then work precisely and methodically as you choose the best product and processing time to achieve the desired result. A pre-service strand test is crucial to success.

Procedure

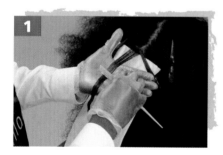

1 Once you have chosen a product strength, complete a strand test. Slip on gloves and carefully follow the manufacturer's application instructions, test a small section of hair from the back of the head. This test will tell you more about the hair's condition, including whether it is weak, strong, dry, or oily. It will also tell you if you have chosen the correct relaxer strength and help you determine the proper processing time, as well as which take-home products to recommend.

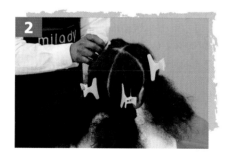

2 When you are ready to proceed with the service, divide the client's hair into four sections, from center of the forehead to the center of the nape, and from ear to ear. Clip each section out of the way.

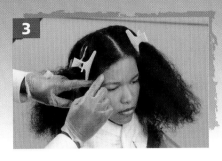

3 Put on a pair of gloves if you have removed the pair used for the test strand and apply a protective cream around the entire hairline.

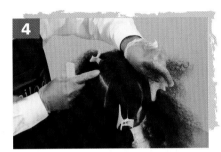

4 If the manufacturer's directions indicate the scalp should be protected, work through each of the four sections taking narrow, ½-inch (1.25 cm) partings and applying a protective base cream to the scalp.

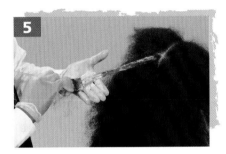

5 Next, take a ½- to 1-inch (1.25 to 2.5 cm) horizontal parting at the top of the back left section. (Base the parting's size on the hair's density.) Brush the relaxing product onto the parting, working ¼- to ½-inch (.6 to 1.25 cm) off the scalp. Natural body heat from the scalp will extend the relaxer toward the scalp. Stop 1½ to 2 inches (3.75 to 5 cm) before the porous ends, particularly if they are damaged. Apply the relaxer to both the top and underside of the parting and then fold the strand up, out of the way.

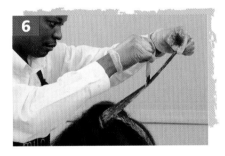

6 Move down, take another ½-inch (1.25 cm) horizontal parting and repeat the application. Work through the section quickly and methodically, brushing the product onto both sides of the partings.

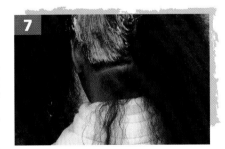

7 Stop before the fragile nape hairline; it will be done later.

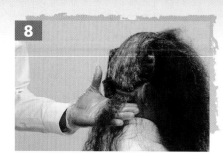

8 Move to the opposite back section and repeat the procedure.

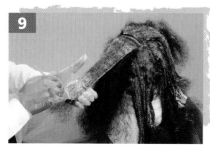

9 Before moving onto the top sections, carefully move folded-up strands back in place so that they hang straight down. Then move to the top left and top right sections. Use horizontal partings and work quickly and methodically.

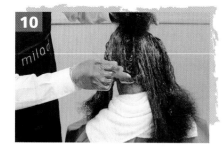

10 When the application is completed, go back and apply the relaxer to the fragile nape and front hairline. The entire application should take 6 to 10 minutes.

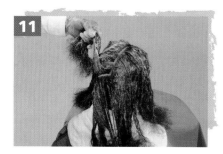

11 Once the application is completed, return to your starting point in back and cross-check your application. Keep the partings straight as you check for missed areas. Apply more product if needed.

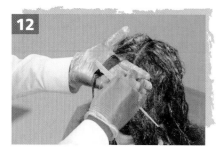

12 Return to the first parting to which you applied the relaxer, and begin smoothing the hair. Take the parting in the palm of one hand and smooth it by pressing from top to bottom with the back of the comb. Using the comb allows even pressure and greater control than using your fingers.

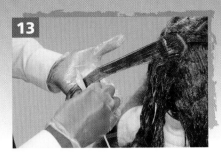

13 If you applied the relaxer by using horizontal partings, smooth the strands using diagonal partings. This avoids splits or obvious parts. Keep the partings as straight as possible and work quickly and methodically following the same sequence you used to apply the relaxer. Work through each section in this manner.

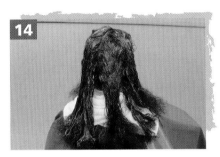

14 When all the sections have been smoothed, process according to manufacturer's directions.

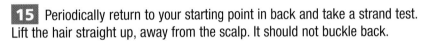

15 Periodically return to your starting point in back and take a strand test. Lift the hair straight up, away from the scalp. It should not buckle back.

16 Another way to perform a test strand is to push the hair into a wave—if processing is completed the hair should not create an S-shape. Continue taking strand tests every few minutes.

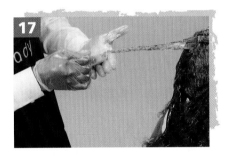

17 During the last few minutes of processing, extend the relaxer as close to the scalp as you can get without touching it with the product. Also extend it through the ends.

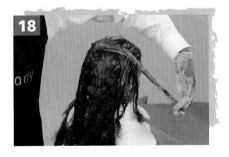

18 The entire process, including smoothing, should take 15 to 17 minutes, or 18 to 20 minutes for coarse, resistant hair.

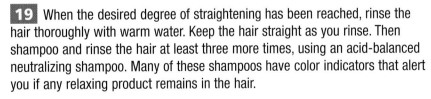

19 When the desired degree of straightening has been reached, rinse the hair thoroughly with warm water. Keep the hair straight as you rinse. Then shampoo and rinse the hair at least three more times, using an acid-balanced neutralizing shampoo. Many of these shampoos have color indicators that alert you if any relaxing product remains in the hair.

Part 2: Chemical Texture Services

Consultation and Application for a Sodium Hydroxide Relaxer on Virgin Hair continued

20 Once rinsing is completed, towel-blot and condition the hair following the manufacturer's directions. Cut and style as desired.

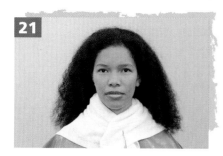

21 Before Sodium Hydroxide Relaxer on Virgin Hair Procedure service.

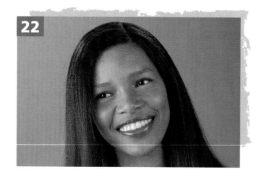

22 After Sodium Hydroxide Relaxer on Virgin Hair Procedure service. The finished look shows smooth, shiny, straightened hair that can be styled for a variety of looks with roller setting, iron curling, or other techniques.

Create

Apply this technique to different hair lengths, colors, and textures for almost endless possibilities.

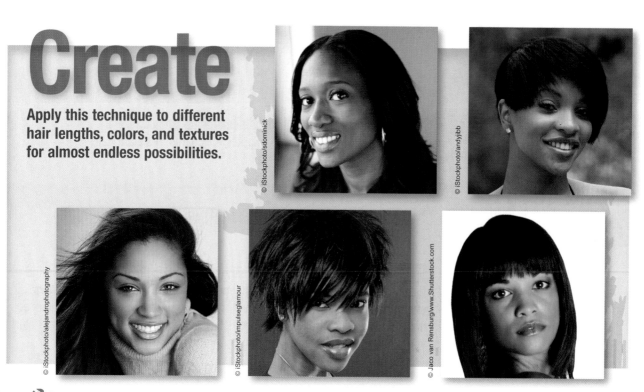

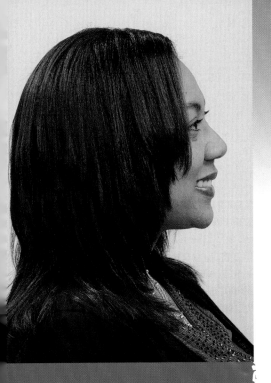

Retouch with a Sodium Hydroxide Relaxer

Implements and Materials

You will need all of the following implements, materials, and supplies:

- **Acid-balanced neutralizing shampoo**
- **Bowl and applicator brush**
- **Conditioner**
- **Disposable gloves**
- **Hard rubber comb**
- **Hydroxide neutralizer**
- **Hydroxide relaxer**
- **Plastic clips**
- **Protective base cream**
- **Chemical cape**
- **Spray bottle**
- **Styling comb**
- **Timer**
- **Towels**

Overview

Six to eight weeks after a client has received a sodium hydroxide relaxer service, new hair will have grown in, and this new growth will have the same textural characteristics as the hair did before straightening. To make this new hair just as straight as the rest of the hair requires a relaxer. Applying permanent relaxer to the new growth only is called a retouch.

Always use a product that is compatible with the initial relaxing product. Sodium hydroxide relaxers can only be retouched with sodium hydroxide products. If the relaxer was performed at home or at another salon, choose a product strength based on elasticity and porosity tests. These tests should be performed during every retouch service, whether or not you performed the initial application. The condition of the hair and scalp can easily change within a few weeks.

Retouch with a Sodium Hydroxide Relaxer
continued

Procedure

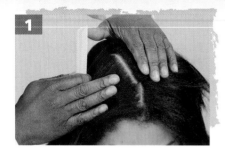

1   Examine the scalp for abrasions or any contraindications. Only proceed if there are no scalp-sensitivity issues. Perform an elasticity test on various areas of the head. Start at the back crest of the head and take one hair strand. Hold the strand of hair firmly at the scalp and wrap it around one of your fingers to gently stretch it. If the hair stretches and does not return to its original form, or breaks, this hair has poor elasticity and should not be relaxed at this time. (Normal, dry hair stretches 20 percent before breaking.)

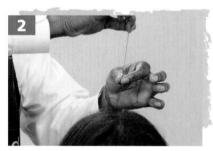

2   Perform a porosity test. Hold five or seven strands up by the ends. Run your fingers from the opposite hand down the strands. If your fingers do not glide down easily or if more than a few strands bunch up at the bottom, the hair is porous. This test will help you select the correct product strength.

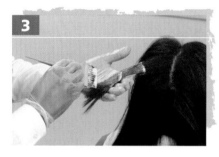

3   Once you have chosen a product, perform a complete test strand. Slip on gloves and carefully follow the manufacturer's application instructions, using a small section of hair from the back of the head. This test will tell you more about the hair's condition, including whether it is weak, strong, dry, or oily. It will also tell you if you have chosen the correct relaxer strength and help you determine the proper processing time, as well as which take-home products to recommend.

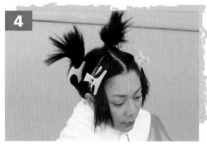

4   When you are ready to proceed with the service, divide the client's hair into four sections by parting from the center of the forehead to the center of the nape, and from ear to ear. Clip sections up to keep them out of the way.

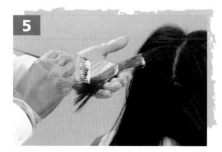

5   Apply a protective cream to the entire hairline. Put gloves on both hands if you have removed the ones used for the test strand. Working through each section in ¼-inch (.6 cm) partings, apply the protective cream to the scalp (unless you are using a no-base product). To prevent overlap, also apply a protective conditioner to the previously relaxed hair.

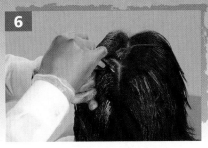

6 Begin the bowl-and-brush application in the most resistant area, usually at the back of the head. Then take a ¼-inch to ½-inch (.6 to 1.25 cm) horizontal parting and apply the relaxer to the regrowth, up to the previously relaxed hair. Apply the relaxer on both the top and underside of the parting. Do not touch the scalp with the relaxer, stay about ¼-inch (.6 cm) off the scalp. Natural body heat will extend the product toward the scalp.

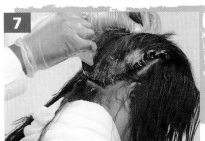

7 Continue applying the relaxer, using the same procedure and working your way down the section toward the hairline. Complete both back sections. If the hairline regrowth is fragile leave it for last.

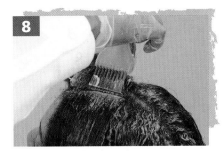

8 Complete both top sections. Apply the relaxer to the most resistant areas first as you repeat the retouch application.

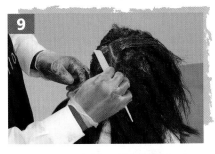

9 Quickly cross-check your work and reapply the product to any missed areas. Apply relaxer to the fragile hairline last. Then return to your starting point and begin smoothing the regrowth area with the back of the comb. Press the regrowth; do not comb through it. Work through each section taking the same-sized partings used for the application—following the application sequence—as you smooth each parting.

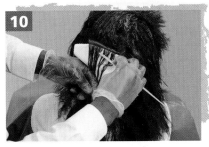

10 Process according to the manufacturer's directions. As soon as the smoothing procedure is completed, take a strand test. Continue to perform periodic strand tests during processing until the desired degree of curl reduction is achieved. The hair should not buckle back when lifted straight out from the head or create an S-shape when pushed upward. During the last few minutes of processing, extend the relaxer down to the scalp without touching it.

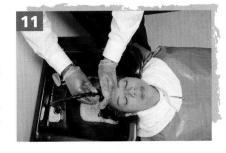

11 When processing is completed, rinse the hair thoroughly with warm water to remove all traces of the relaxer. As you rinse, keep the hair straight. Then shampoo and rinse the hair at least three more times with an acid-balanced neutralizing shampoo or one with a color indicator. It is essential that all traces of the relaxer be removed from the hair.

© Milady, a part of Cengage Learning. Photography by Gary David Gold.

Part 2: Chemical Texture Services

Retouch with a Sodium Hydroxide Relaxer
continued

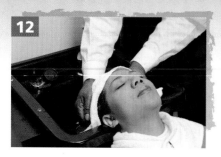

12 Once rinsing is completed, towel-blot and condition the hair following the manufacturer's directions. Cut and style as desired.

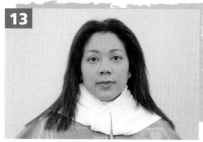

13 Before Retouch with a Sodium Hydroxide Relaxer Procedure service.

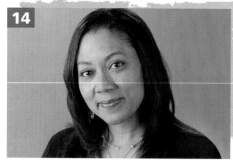

14 After Retouch with a Sodium Hydroxide Relaxer Procedure service. In the finished look, the regrowth now blends beautifully with the previously relaxed hair.

Create

Apply this technique to different hair lengths, colors, and textures for almost endless possibilities.

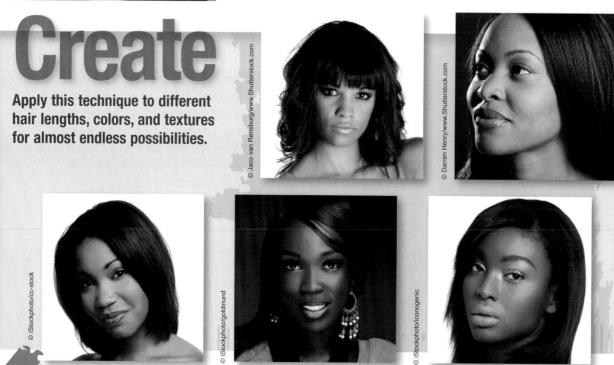

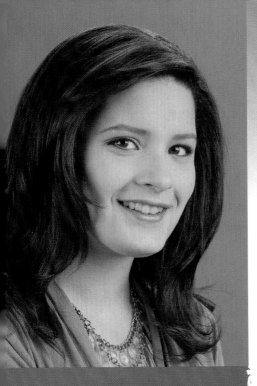

Applying Thio Relaxer to Virgin Hair

Implements and Materials

You will need all of the following implements, materials, and supplies:

- **Bowl and applicator brush**
- **Conditioner**
- **Disposable gloves**
- **Hard rubber comb**
- **Plastic clips**
- **Pre-neutralizing conditioner**
- **Protective base cream**
- **Chemical cape**
- **Spray bottle**
- **Styling comb**
- **Thio neutralizer**
- **Thio relaxer**
- **Timer**
- **Towels**

Overview

The application steps for thio relaxers are the same as those used for sodium hydroxide relaxers; it is the neutralization steps that are different. Once the thio relaxer is rinsed from the hair, it is thoroughly blotted. Then a neutralizer, which is an oxidizing agent, is applied. The oxidation reaction rebuilds the bonds that were broken and a new, straighter texture is achieved.

Never use a thio relaxer on hair that has been exposed to sodium hydroxide. Also, if the hair is to be colored with a permanent haircoloring product, this should be done 2 weeks after thio relaxing. If you color the hair first, the thio relaxer will lighten the haircolor.

Procedure

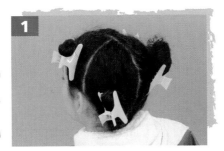

1 Part the hair into four sections, from the center of the front hairline to the center of the nape, and from ear to ear. Clip the sections up to keep them out of the way.

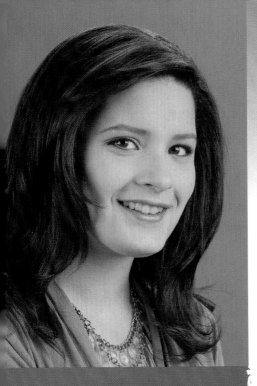

Applying Thio Relaxer to Virgin Hair
continued

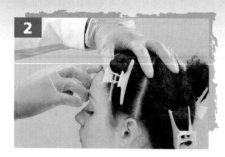

2   Put gloves on both hands and apply protective base cream to the hairline and ears. Option: Take ¼-inch to ½-inch (.6 to 1.25 cm) horizontal partings and apply a protective base cream to the entire scalp. Always follow the manufacturer's directions and the procedures approved by your instructor.

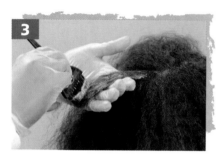

3   Begin application in the most resistant area, usually at the back of the head. Make ¼-inch to ½-inch (.6 to 1.25 cm) horizontal partings and apply the relaxer to the top of the strand first, then to the underside. Apply the relaxer with an applicator brush, with the back of the comb, or with your fingers. Apply relaxer ¼-inch to ½-inch (.6 to 1.25 cm) away from the scalp and up to the porous ends. To avoid scalp irritation, do not allow the relaxer to touch the scalp until the last few minutes of processing.

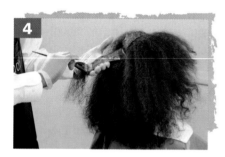

4   Continue applying the relaxer, working your way down the section toward the hairline.

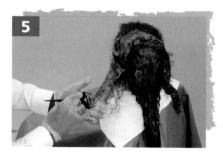

5   Continue the same application procedure with the remaining sections. Finish the most resistant sections first.

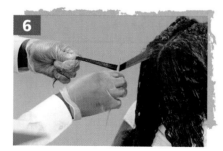

6   After the relaxer has been applied to all sections, use the back of the comb or your hands to smooth each section. Never comb the relaxer through the hair.

Part 2: Chemical Texture Services

7 Process according to the manufacturer's directions. Perform periodic strand tests. Always follow manufacturer's processing and timing directions.

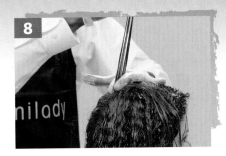

8 During the last few minutes of processing, work the relaxer on both the top and underside of the strand down to the scalp and through the ends of the hair, using additional relaxer as needed. Carefully smooth all sections using an applicator brush, your fingers, or the back of the comb.

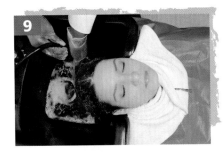

9 Rinse thoroughly with warm water to remove all traces of the relaxer.

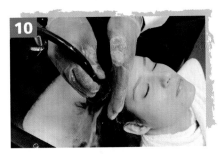

10 Be certain all traces of relaxer are removed from the hair. Optional: Apply the pre-neutralizing conditioner and comb it through to the ends of the hair. Leave it on for approximately five minutes and then rinse. Always follow the manufacturer's directions and the procedures approved by your instructor.

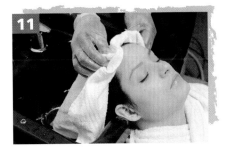

11 Blot excess water from the hair.

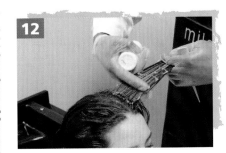

12 Apply thio neutralizer in ¼- to ½-inch (.6 to 1.25 cm) sections throughout the hair and smooth with your hands or the back of the comb.

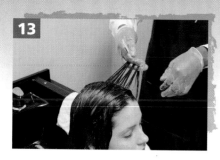

13 Process the neutralizer according to the manufacturer's directions.

14 Rinse thoroughly, condition, and style.

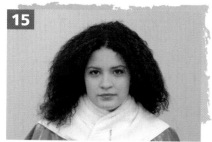

15 Before Applying Thio Relaxer to Virgin Hair Procedure service.

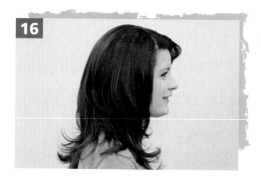

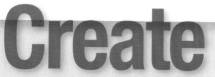

16 After Applying Thio Relaxer to Virgin Hair Procedure service.

Create

Apply this technique to different hair lengths, colors, and textures for almost endless possibilities.

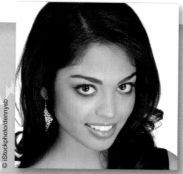

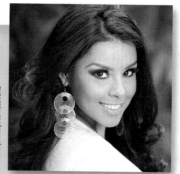

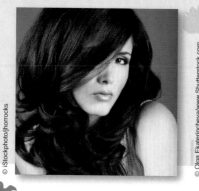

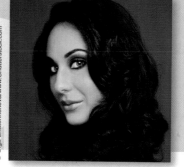

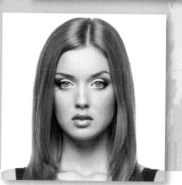

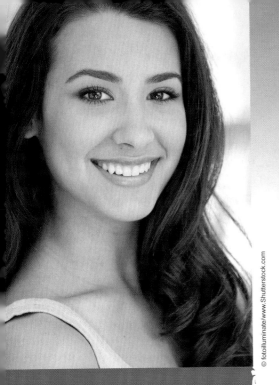

Thio Relaxer Retouch

Implements and Materials

You will need all of the following implements, materials, and supplies:

- **Bowl and applicator brush**
- **Conditioner**
- **Disposable gloves**
- **Hard rubber comb**
- **Plastic clips**
- **Pre-neutralizing conditioner**
- **Protective base cream**
- **Chemical cape**
- **Spray bottle**
- **Styling comb**
- **Thio neutralizer**
- **Thio relaxer**
- **Timer**
- **Towels**

Overview

Performing a thio relaxer retouch is very similar to performing a sodium hydroxide relaxer retouch. Only the neutralization procedure is different. When performing the retouch, make certain the initial procedure was done with a thio-based product.

Even if you performed the initial thio relaxing service, conduct a thorough hair and scalp analysis prior to the retouch. The hair's condition can change within 4 to 6 weeks; only proceed if there are no contraindications.

Procedure

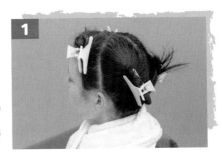

1 Divide the hair into four sections, from the center of the front hairline to the center of the nape, and from ear to ear. Clip sections up to keep them out of the way.

Thio Relaxer Retouch continued

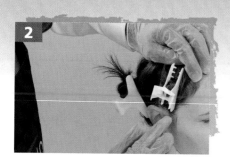

2 Apply a protective base cream to the hairline and ears, unless you are using a no-base relaxing product. Put gloves on both hands. Option: Take ¼-inch to ½-inch (.6 to 1.25 cm) horizontal partings and apply protective base cream to the entire scalp.

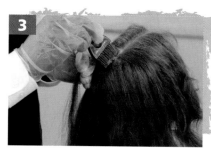

3 Begin application of the relaxer in the most resistant area, usually at the back of the head. Make ¼-inch to ½-inch (.6 to 1.25 cm) horizontal partings and apply the relaxer to both sides of the regrowth area. Apply the relaxer as close to the scalp as possible, but do not touch the scalp with the relaxer. Only allow the relaxer to touch the scalp itself during the last few minutes of processing. To avoid overprocessing or breakage, do not overlap the relaxer onto the previously relaxed hair.

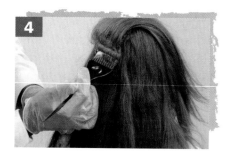

4 Continue applying the relaxer, using the same procedure and working your way down the section toward the hairline.

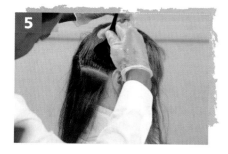

5 Continue the same application procedure with the remaining sections, finishing the most resistant sections first.

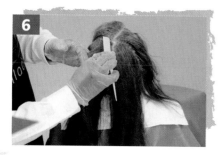

6 After the relaxer has been applied to all sections, use the back of the comb, the applicator brush, or your hands to smooth each section.

Part 2: Chemical Texture Services

7 Process according to the manufacturer's directions. Perform periodic strand tests. Processing usually takes less than 20 minutes at room temperature. Always follow the manufacturer's processing directions.

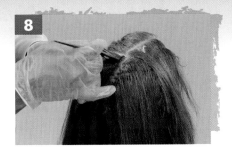

8 During the last few minutes of processing, gently work the relaxer down to the scalp.

9 If the ends of the hair need additional relaxing, work the relaxer through to the ends for the last few minutes of processing. Do not relax ends during each retouch; doing this will cause overprocessing. Option: A cream conditioner may be applied to relaxed ends to protect from overprocessing caused by overlapping.

10 Rinse thoroughly with warm water to remove all traces of the relaxer.

11 Make certain all traces of the relaxer have been removed from the hair. Optional: Before neutralizing you may wish to apply the pre-neutralizing conditioner and comb it through to the ends of the hair. Leave it on for approximately 5 minutes and then rinse. Always follow the manufacturer's directions and the procedures approved by your instructor.

12 Blot excess water from hair.

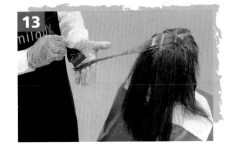

13 Apply thio neutralizer in ¼- to ½-inch (.6 to 1.25 cm) sections throughout the hair and smooth with your hands or the back of the comb.

14 Process the neutralizer according to the manufacturer's directions.

15 Rinse thoroughly, condition, and style.

Thio Relaxer Retouch continued

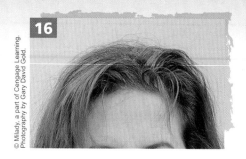

16 Before Thio Relaxer Retouch Procedure service.

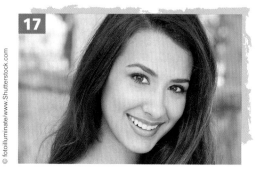

17 After Thio Relaxer Retouch Procedure service.

Create

Apply this technique to different hair lengths, colors, and textures for almost endless possibilities.

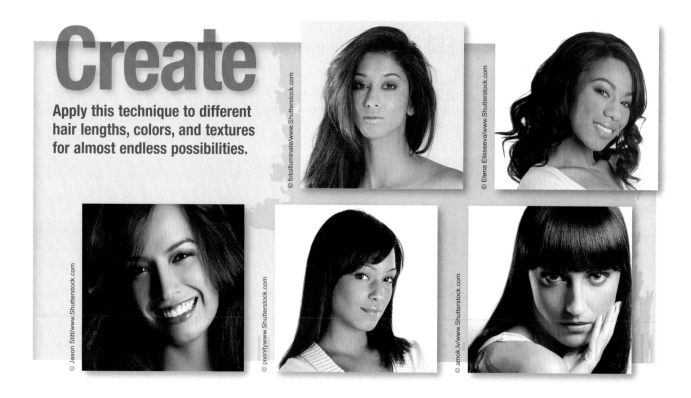

Part 2: Chemical Texture Services

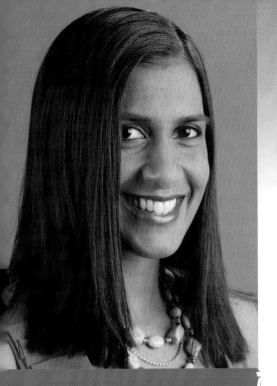

Thermal Reconditioning (Straightening) Treatment

Implements and Materials

You will need all of the following implements, materials, and supplies:

- **Professional thermal reconditioning (straightening) treatment product system including companion shampoo, conditioner, and hair treatment**
- **Flat iron that reaches up to 450 degrees Fahrenheit (232 C)**
- **Professional blowdryer**
- **Round blowdrying brush**
- **Wide-toothed comb**
- **Bowl and applicator brush**
- **Disposable gloves**
- **Plastic clips**
- **Chemical cape**
- **Styling comb**
- **Timer**
- **Towels**

Overview

Thermal Reconditioning (Straightening) Treatments should not be done on certain hair types, including lightened or "bleached" hair, hair that is tightly coiled or extremely curly, and hair that has been previously relaxed with a sodium hydroxide product. Because the service uses a thioglycolate product, it is not compatible with sodium hydroxide. Thermal Reconditioning is considered a specialty, and most manufacturers require certification in their particular procedure. Thermal Straightening, done incorrectly, can result in hair breakage.

After the service, hair should not be colored for at least 2 weeks. The service combines a thioglycolate product, heat from a flat iron, and mechanical stress to achieve the desired results. Because you must get close to the scalp with the flat iron, the hair must be at least 4-inches (10 cm) long. The procedure takes 4 to 6 hours or more, depending on the hair's density and texture. To speed the procedure, many salons have two stylists work on a single client.

Some manufacturers add extra steps to protect the hair at specific stages. Usually, after the service, the hair must remain untouched for 72 hours—no ponytails, showers, or workouts.

These systems differ in many ways. What remains the same is that you apply a thio-based solution to very fine sections of hair, then process, rinse, and blowdry it completely. Next, the same fine sections of hair are flat ironed by making several passes with the flat iron. The hair is then neutralized; this step is sometimes called conditioning or bonding, depending on the manufacturer. If a neutralizer is used, the hair is then rinsed before it is blown dry. Always follow the manufacturer's directions completely.

© Milady, a part of Cengage Learning. Photography by Gary David Gold.

Thermal Reconditioning (Straightening) Treatment continued

Procedure

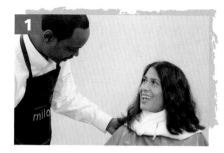

1 Consult with the client regarding her hair's history of chemical applications and her desired results.

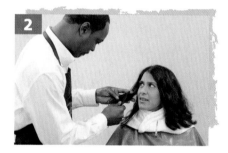

2 Check the hair for porosity. If the hair is porous, the formula will penetrate faster. Often, a protein conditioner is applied to equalize porosity.

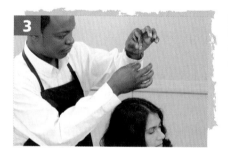

3 Perform a strand test to determine the hair's tensile strength. Also check for any damage, and observe the curl pattern for looser or tighter areas. Do not proceed if there are any contraindications.

4 Rinse the hair with warm water. If the manufacturer allows, lightly shampoo and rinse completely. Towel-dry the hair. (Some manufacturers require you to partially blowdry the hair at this stage.)

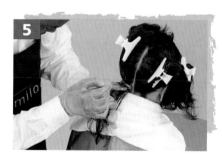

5 Divide the hair into quadrants. Begin at the lower left side, take a ¼- to ½-inch (.6 to 1.25 cm) wide horizontal parting and apply the thio solution to the hair. Work ¼ to ½ inch (.6 to 1.25 cm) away from the scalp to the ends. Do not apply the product to the scalp. Apply it to both the top and underside of the parting. In some cases the solution will be a cream and in other instances it may be a gel-like substance applied with an applicator brush; in others, it will be a spray-on product that you work through with gloved hands. Keep the hair as straight as possible during the application and processing steps.

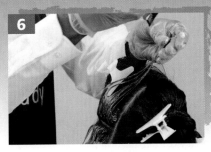

6 Work up the section, taking fine partings and repeating the application procedure. Some manufacturers recommend smoothing with the back of the comb; do not smooth through unless the manufacturer allows. Even then, if you comb the hair, only comb through every three partings as one—do not comb partings individually.

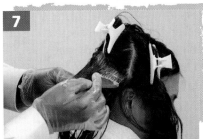

7 When you reach the top, move to the next section and repeat the application procedure.

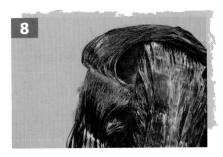

8 Work through each section in the same manner, systematically applying the solution.

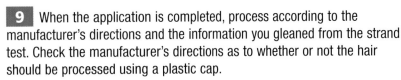

9 When the application is completed, process according to the manufacturer's directions and the information you gleaned from the strand test. Check the manufacturer's directions as to whether or not the hair should be processed using a plastic cap.

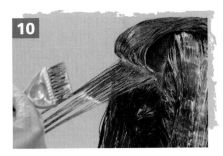

10 During the last few minutes apply the thio solution to the scalp area, and then begin taking strand tests after 5 minutes. Processing could take as long as half an hour depending on the hair type, curl pattern, and manufacturer product. Pay close attention to areas where curl was the strongest. If necessary, the formula can often be reapplied to these areas. Continue to strand test every 3 to 5 minutes.

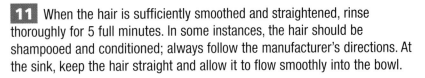

11 When the hair is sufficiently smoothed and straightened, rinse thoroughly for 5 full minutes. In some instances, the hair should be shampooed and conditioned; always follow the manufacturer's directions. At the sink, keep the hair straight and allow it to flow smoothly into the bowl.

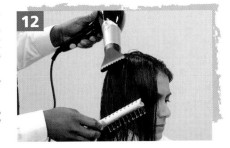

12 Apply a heat protector or protein solution, based on manufacturer's instructions. Then blowdry the hair, being careful not to bend or clip it. Again, depending on the manufacturer, you may dry the hair completely or partially.

Thermal Reconditioning (Straightening) Treatment continued

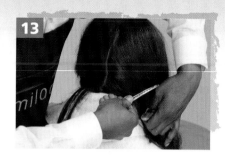

13 Resection the hair into quadrants, which will be flat ironed by taking fine partings within each section. The flat ironing or pressing procedure determines how smooth and straight the results will be. Iron temperature is very important to results; always follow the manufacturer's guidelines. In general, professionals advise never exceeding 356 degrees Fahrenheit (180 C); some manufacturers recommend temperatures as high as 428 degrees Fahrenheit (220 C), and temperature limits are far lower for color-treated or damaged hair: 284 degrees Fahrenheit (140 C).

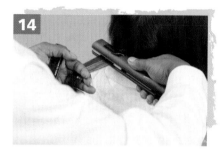

14 Begin the flat ironing procedure at the bottom of the back left side, using extremely fine subsections that are about ⅛-inch (.3 cm) wide.

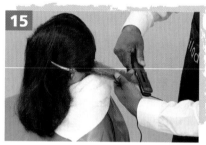

15 Starting at the nape and holding the hair at a 90-degree angle, use the flat iron to gently press the parting in a downward motion. First, work from the scalp area to the midlenghts. Make two to three passes with the iron, then repeat. Get as close to the scalp as possible. Use a fine-toothed comb to control and direct the hair. Then press all the way from the scalp area to the ends two to three more times. Some manufacturers instruct you to first press two to three partings from the scalp area to the midshaft, and then combine the partings and press from the scalp area to the ends two to three times. Always follow the manufacturer's directions.

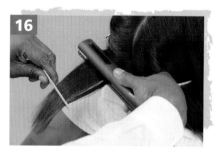

16 Work up the section, repeating the pressing procedure with fine partings. Each parting should be flat ironed several times. Take time and care—this is a tedious but very important task.

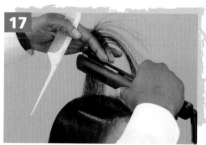

17 Working through the quadrants clockwise around the head, complete each section in the same manner. When you reach the top, lift partings straight up from the base to get close to the scalp. Keep the hair straight, as you pull the iron upward.

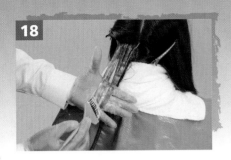
18

18 Once the flat ironing is completed, put on gloves and part the hair again into four sections. Apply the neutralizer from scalp to the ends of the partings. Some manufacturers use a brush and bowl method, others advise different methods such as misting on a leave-in conditioner at this point and proceeding to blowdrying. If using a bowl and brush, work in narrow partings from the nape up, using a downward motion. Work through all the sections. Then process according to the manufacturer's directions.

19 If you applied a neutralizer or bonding agent, rinse thoroughly and condition according to the manufacturer's instructions.

20 Blowdry the hair in the same direction it was flat ironed. Most manufacturers do not allow shampooing for 72 hours. Always follow the manufacturer's instructions meticulously.

21 Before Thermal Reconditioning (Straightening) Treatment Procedure service.

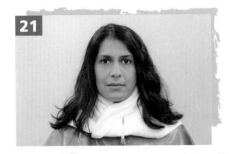
21

22 After Thermal Reconditioning (Straightening) Treatment Procedure service. In the finished look, the newly straightened hair is shiny and healthy looking. Always advise the client on home-care, based on the manufacturer's specific instructions. Most manufacturers also have home-care systems for their products.

22

Create

Apply this technique to different hair lengths, colors, and textures for almost endless possibilities.

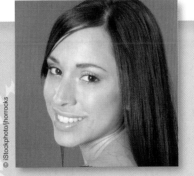
© iStockphoto/jhorrocks

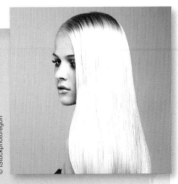
© iStockphoto/egorr

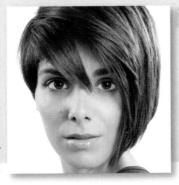
© iStockphoto/ridofrance

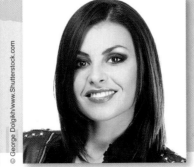
© George Dolgikh/www.Shutterstock.com

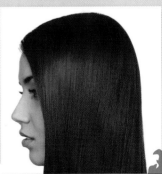
© Andriy Goncharenko / www.Shutterstock.com